Please return to: _____ UK

D0567810

pilates
body in motion

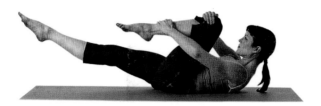

pilates
body in motion

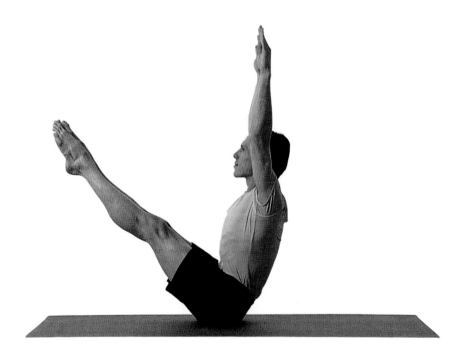

ALYCEA UNGARO
PHOTOGRAPHY BY RUSSELL SADUR

A Dorling Kindersley Book

LONDON, NEW YORK, MUNICH,
MELBOURNE, AND DELHI

For Emma and Estelle

Project Editor Irene Lyford **Designer** Kenny Grant
Senior Editor Jennifer Jones **Art Editor** Sara Robin
Managing Editor Gillian Roberts **Senior Art Editor** Karen Sawyer
Category Publisher Mary-Clare Jerram **Art Director** Tracy Killick
DTP Louise Waller **Production** Louise Daly

First edition published in Great Britain in 2002
by Dorling Kindersley Limited
80 Strand, London WC2R 0RL
A Penguin Company

Copyright © 2002 Dorling Kindersley
Text Copyright © 2002 Alycea Ungaro

2 4 6 8 10 9 7 5 3

All rights reserved. No part of this publication may be reproduced,
stored in a retrieval system, or transmitted in any form or by any means,
electronic, mechanical, photocopying or otherwise, without the prior
written permission of the copyright owners.

A CIP catalogue record for this book is available from The British Library

ISBN 0 7513 3691 2

Colour reproduction by Colorscan, Singapore
Printed and bound in Spain by Artes Grafias

See our complete catalogue at
www.dk.com

CONTENTS

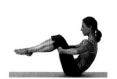 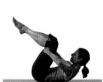 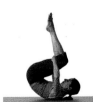 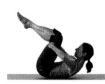 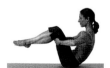

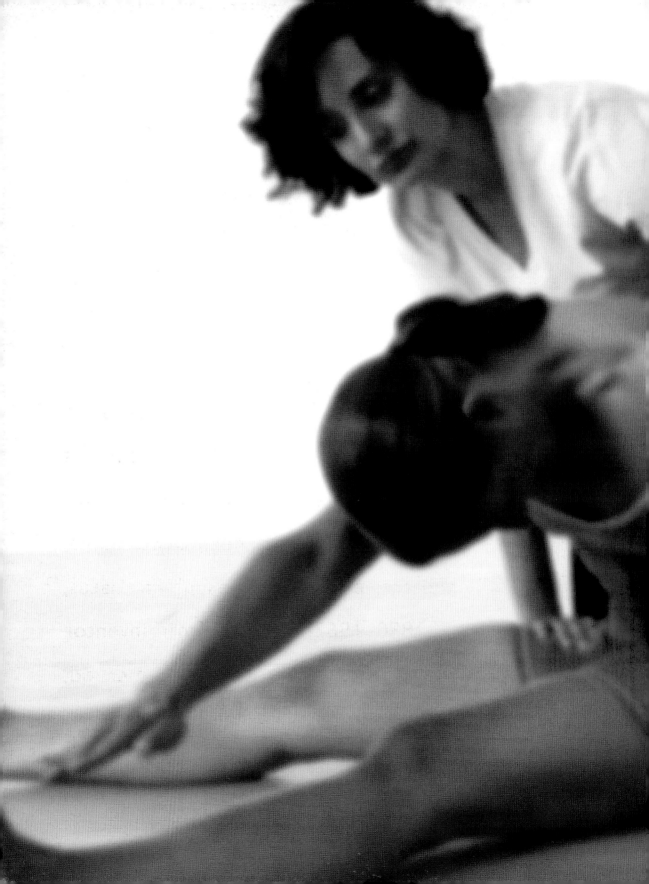

INTRODUCTION

Pilates (pih-lah-teez) *n.* 1. A movement system that uses spring-driven machines as well as a series of floor exercises to increase strength, flexibility, stamina, and concentration. 2. Joseph H. Pilates, 1880–1967, noted German inventor of the Pilates exercise method, originally called "Contrology".

DEFINING PILATES

Dozens of times each day, in the course of teaching students and treating patients, I am asked to define Pilates. Yet, as I approach my twentieth year of experience with the method, the question still finds me struggling for a simple phrase that encapsulates and embodies all that Pilates is.

Pilates is exercise. It is a physical training regimen based on the body in its most natural state – in motion. Pilates is an art form, similar to martial arts or dance, in that it must be worked to perfection on a daily basis. Pilates is a physical science. It is a technique so precise and so concentrated that its results remain with you forever. Pilates is all of these things – and yet none of these definitions really fully explain it.

As I fumbled for the perfect words to commit to paper, it suddenly occurred to me that how I feel about Pilates or how I myself define it is less important than how you, the reader, experience it: My task is to inspire you to try it for yourself. To that end, I will stop struggling to define

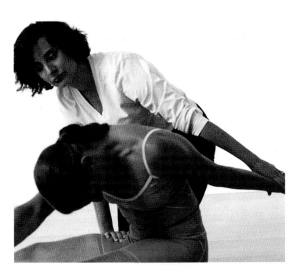

The Pilates method is traditionally performed in one-to-one training sessions. In this way, instructors are best able to tailor the material and the focus of the session to the individual needs of each student's body.

it and instead leave it to you to establish your own definition, not by simply reading about it or listening to someone else, but by physically experiencing it.

Pilates: Body in Motion is designed as a guide and a reference. My aim is to present the method to you in a clear and concise way and, in so doing, to instruct, guide, and facilitate your independent mastery of the Pilates technique in its purest form.

WHO WAS JOSEPH PILATES?

Only a few individuals each century have the ability to challenge conventional beliefs. Whether their field is mathematics, literature, or choreography, these visionaries are so ahead of their time that their ideas and work are astonishingly refreshing and contemporary, even decades later. Such is the case with Joseph H. Pilates, who was born in Germany in 1880.

A sickly childhood led Pilates to pioneer his unique training system, with which he hoped to rid his students of all physical limitations. Inspired by both Eastern and Western philosophies, he combined the mental focus and specific breathing of yoga with the physicality of gymnastics and other sports to create something entirely new.

Early Influences

Germany in the early twentieth century was a hub of dance and exercise development. In addition to his own studies, Pilates was clearly influenced by the other exercise enthusiasts of his time, in particular Eugen Sandow. A fitness pioneer and the darling of royalty, Sandow enjoyed widespread recognition as a bodybuilder and exercise professional and used his popularity to advocate mandatory fitness for children. Following in his footsteps, Pilates championed what he termed an "established physical culture". His great desire was to see his method practised daily by children in schools worldwide.

A Move to New York

In 1926, Pilates came under pressure from Wilhelm II to teach his fitness programme to the new German Army. As a committed pacifist, he promptly left for the United States. Having been involved with the dance community in Germany, it seemed natural for him to introduce his system to the dance and drama capital of the United States – New York City. On the sea crossing to America, Joseph met a nurse named Clara. They eventually married and opened a gym in the building that housed the New York City Ballet. The city embraced Pilates and, as more and more people discovered the method, Pilates devoted himself to further cultivating his system of Contrology. In an effort to bring his method to the masses, Pilates published *Return to Life Through Contrology* – a book devoted to the mat exercises. After his death in 1967, Joseph Pilates' work was carried on primarily by his wife, who is remembered for her wonderful touch and unique ability to impart the essential quality of each movement.

The Pilates method has finally earned its rightful place among the ranks of established exercise systems. Today, more than three decades after his death and nearly a century after his arrival in the United States, Joseph Pilates' work is more popular and accessible than ever.

THE EVOLUTION OF EXERCISE

There are hundreds of fitness techniques, and new methods crop up every day. Still, fitness eludes most people as they struggle to remain either interested in or dedicated to a specific exercise programme. For many, exercise becomes painful and boring drudgery.

In primitive societies, exercise was obtained primarily through hunting and gathering. Our ancestors had physically to overcome huge obstacles in order to eat. Can you imagine early man not being motivated enough

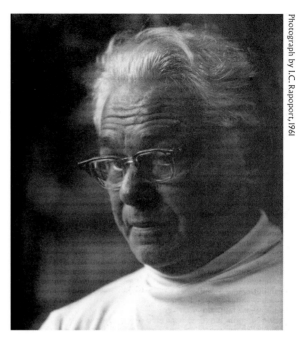

Photograph by I.C. Rapoport, 1961

Joseph Pilates was born in 1880 in Dusseldorf, Germany. He devoted his life to the study of physical education, becoming an accomplished diver, skier, boxer, and gymnast before developing his own exercise system. He continued to teach and refine his method until his death in 1967.

to secure food – or too tired to go on with the hunt? Yet this is the situation in which you may often find yourself with respect to your own exercise routine.

Fitness is no longer a means to an end. In our civilized world, physical conditioning is not necessary for survival. Our survival skills often require no more than lining up at the supermarket – an activity that exercises neither the mind nor the body.

"Man's inherited birthright is physical perfection."

As a result, exercise has become an institution that is both structured and scheduled. To the human body, which has evolved to conserve energy for fight or flight, this condition is unnatural.

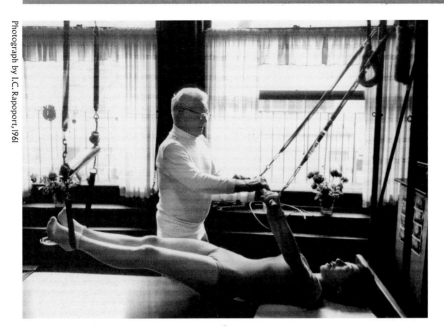

Photograph by I.C. Rapoport, 1961

Joseph Pilates instructs a pupil on the "Cadillac", one of a range of specialized training apparatus that he developed. Here, Mr Pilates guides the student through a beginner level exercise called the "Breathing" – an example of over 100 exercises performed on the Cadillac.

Given our lifestyles, the incentive to be fit must come in other forms. Greater self-esteem, better health, and longevity are all sound reasons to begin a fitness regime. But the best stimulus is the exercise itself, which, ideally, is enjoyable, engaging, and invigorating. These are the basic elements with which Joseph Pilates infused his discipline.

The very structure of the Pilates method requires mental focus, a process that forces your muscles to respond more quickly to training. Rather than performing monotonous and reflexive repetitions, you will carefully execute a limited number of compound movements with an eye towards perfecting every possible detail. By integrating body and mind, you will achieve an effective, efficient, and balanced workout.

BODY MAINTENANCE

I attended my first Pilates class in 1982. I had suffered an ankle injury while a student at the School of American Ballet and my teachers suggested I practise Pilates while I was unable to dance. My first session was overwhelming: I was led from one piece of apparatus to the next like a child at a playground. While the fundamentals were lost on me (all I wished for was a speedy recovery), I had an

instinctive feeling that there was something very valuable about this system. I returned for more instruction, curious as to how this abdominal workout was going to help my ankle. I didn't realize that I was being realigned and symmetrically strengthened. Ultimately, I did return to ballet class and, as my career progressed, so did my injuries. At each impasse, I found myself running to Pilates to keep in shape and hasten recovery. It was not until I was dancing professionally that I realized I should be doing Pilates for maintenance and not just as a fitness substitute.

Pilates as a Way of Life

Life wreaks havoc on our bodies. People grow more and more crooked and imbalanced in the course of daily living. We are right- or left-handed: we swing a golf club or tennis racquet on one side; we carry our shoulder bags and our children on one shoulder or hip. Our routines and habits cause us to consistently overuse some muscles and underuse others. Pilates can be a wonderful antidote to this, providing a workout that will stretch, straighten, and strengthen your body. This method is not a mystical cure-all. Nor should it replace other forms of exercise once you adopt it into your routine. All exercise is good for you. Run, bike, swim, walk – and do Pilates. Pilates will enhance and complement your regular activities to help you look better, perform better, and, above all, feel better.

PILATES TODAY

Pilates today has become a bit of a hotchpotch. Like any other physical system, it is vulnerable to interpretation and embellishment that reflect the experiences of the practitioner. There are infinite styles and breeds, from rehabilitative Pilates to Pilates on a ball. What matters most is that you enjoy your workout and that you get results. What I am presenting here is the closest thing we have to the original method. There have been minor changes over the last 30 years as science advances its understanding of the human body but, despite these adaptations, the brilliance and simplicity of the system remain intact and available to everyone.

The Benefits of Pilates

What should you expect from your Pilates workout? First, you should expect to learn an ordered series of exercises that work the entire body from top to bottom. Expect it to be efficient: by decreasing overall repetitions and increasing the work of each motion, you will obtain rapid and long-lasting results. Plan to work rigorously, with no impact to your joints. Prepare to strengthen and stretch your body during every exercise, rotating positions from lying to sitting to kneeling. Ready yourself to activate your mind as you exercise, developing and increasing your awareness of your body. Finally, and perhaps most significantly, expect your workouts to fly by.

To do Pilates "proper" means to work the entire system with all of its components. If at all possible, invest in some one-to-one sessions at a fully equipped studio. There you can experience the equipment and the benefit of a trained instructor's eye. Then take the experience home with you. The matwork is the most accessible part of the method and it can be done virtually anywhere – but there is a price. You must invest your time and energy in order to learn it. Let us begin with the founding principles.

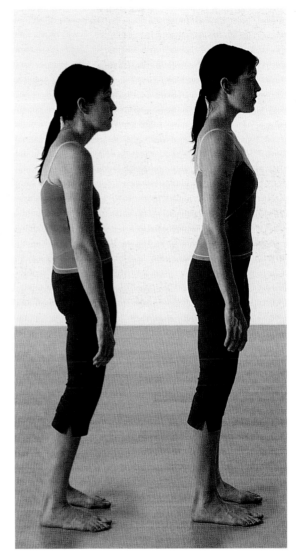

Postural misalignment *(above left)* occurs as a result of poor body mechanics, weakened muscular structures, and reduced muscular endurance. Note the student's stooped posture. The chest muscles are concave and the shoulders are rounded forwards, forcing the hips to shift forwards.

Proper alignment *(above right)* is demonstrated in a healthy, strong spine, by a plumb line through the centre of the body, landing just in front of the ankle. Here the chest remains open and the shoulders are back, allowing the lower body to align properly with the upper body.

PHILOSOPHY OF FORM

Mr Pilates formulated six original principles that will both establish and improve the quality of your workout. These concepts are not limited to Pilates, but can be applied to any exercise, indoors or out, and ultimately to all aspects of your daily life.

Breath

Joseph Pilates wrote: "above all ... learn to breathe correctly." Correct breathing oxygenates the blood and increases circulation. In Pilates, a structured breathing technique is an effective tool that is meant to enhance and ease your movements. Never, under any circumstances, should you stop breathing. As exercises increase in difficulty, you may find yourself holding your breath through the challenging sections As a general rule, we inhale to prepare for a movement and exhale as we execute it, particularly through the more difficult parts. Always breathe deeply and fully, in through the nose and out through the mouth.

Concentration

There are no mindless or careless moments in Pilates. Rather than diverting your attention or allowing your thoughts to wander, focus your mind on the task in hand. During each part of every movement you should be conducting an internal dialogue, directing your body through the exercise. When you can perform a mental checklist during each exercise, you will have begun to master the learning process. Concentrate on what is correct and what is incorrect, and concentrate on improving your form by focusing on every detail.

Control

Joseph Pilates dubbed his method "Contrology" or "The Art of Control". In any physical science, control must be practised and developed. Pilates requires the complete control of your body by your mind. Every motion you perform should be meticulously calculated and planned for. In this way the Pilates method reduces the risk of injury and trains your body for life in the same way that an athlete's training regime prepares them for an event.

Centring

Pilates is often described as "movement flowing out from a strong centre". Your centre is the foundation for all of your movements. No arm or leg gesture occurs without a strong and stable centre. We define the "centre" as the wide band of midsection from your navel around to your lower back, extending from your lower ribs to just below your buttocks. Each and every exercise in this book focuses on strengthening this centre.

The Boomerang, an advanced level exercise, demonstrates the principles of the Pilates method. Each pose shown is simply one part of the exercise that connects to the next, creating a smooth stream of movement. Although it is difficult to imagine the use of *breath* and *flow* from these static pictures, the pupil must use both to successfully perform the movement. The remaining elements of *precision*, *concentration*, *centring*, and *control* , which are required to execute such an exercise, are clearly depicted. The execution of these principles distinguishes Pilates from other exercise systems.

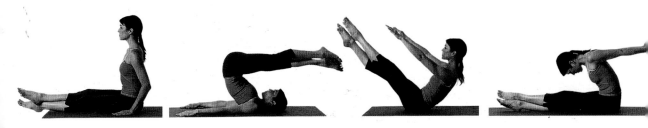

Precision

Precision elevates the benefits of each exercise from superficial to intense. Do not focus simply on completing an exercise but on performing the exercise as perfectly as possible. Apply precision to all aspects of your workout and your body will surely benefit.

> ## "What is balance of body and mind ... conscious control of all muscular movements."

Be precise in your approach, your focus, and your form. It is not the structure of the exercise but the work you put into it that determines your results.

Flow

Flow is one of the principles that distinguishes Pilates from other fitness regimes. Movement is by nature continuous: in daily life, movements are connected to one another and are never fragmented or isolated. In your Pilates workout, concentrate on flow during each individual exercise, but also as you thread the exercises together. Executed this way your workout will improve your balance, control, and coordination, thus preparing your body for the rigorous demands of daily life.

SYNTHESIS AND INTEGRATION

As you begin your study of this method, you may be overwhelmed by how these six principles transform a seemingly basic exercise system into a complex world of motion. Each Pilates exercise is designed to include these elements, but, without an instructor to prompt your memory, your technique may become haphazard and the results unpredictable. To incorporate these founding rules successfully, tackle one concept at a time until it becomes habitual. Begin with the introductory and beginner's programmes and work on infusing each exercise with these principles. Once they become second nature in a small group of exercises, it should be simple to carry over the techniques to the more advanced material.

Spine Stretch Forward This beginner's level exercise (*see pp60–61*) shows the use of the principles in a more basic position. The model employs *precision* and *concentration* to align herself accurately. *Control* is used to avoid collapsing over. *Centring* is exercised as the movement initiates from the centre of the body rather than the limbs. Finally, the student uses her *breath* as she stretches forwards, exhaling all the air before using *flow* to glide back up to a tall upright position.

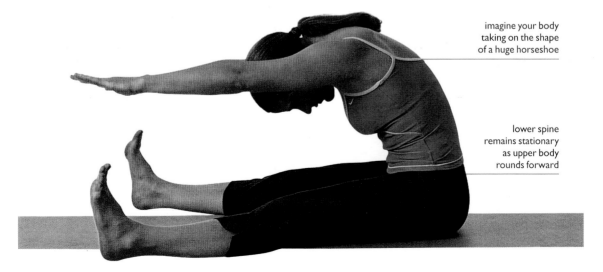

imagine your body taking on the shape of a huge horseshoe

lower spine remains stationary as upper body rounds forward

THE LANGUAGE OF PILATES

There is a vocabulary that is specific to Pilates and certain expressions are repeated time and again. Your goal is to drill these phrases into your mind and into your body so that the words themselves become movements that infiltrate your workout. This section provides a key to the most common phrases.

LATERAL BREATHING

Mr Pilates was asthmatic and therefore was understandably focused on proper breathing. He advocated inhalations that filled the lungs entirely and exhalations that emptied the lungs to the very bottom, cleansing the bloodstream and purifying the body of toxins. The Pilates method as performed today follows a simple breathing technique known as lateral breathing.

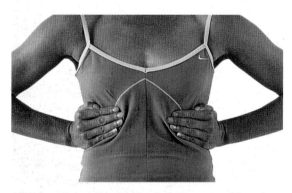

Actively exhale, collapsing the ribs as far as possible and feeling the two sides of your rib cage coming together.

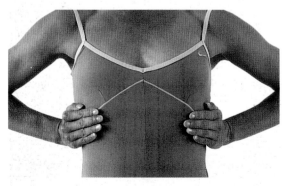

Breathe in, allowing your ribs to push outwards, laterally, into your hands without expanding the belly.

Our lungs lie nestled within our rib cage. As a general rule, women are apical or upper chest breathers, elevating the shoulders and the upper body with each breath. Men tend to be more diaphragmatic breathers, filling the belly with each breath. In Pilates we practise lateral breathing — expanding the ribs sideways with each breath. This technique allows us to hold the abdominals concave and simultaneously keep the upper body relaxed. Before embarking upon this programme, take a few minutes to practise lateral breathing. Follow the instructions provided in the illustrations (*left*).

THE PILATES BOX

The box is your key to proper alignment, which will ensure that the body is training symmetrically and therefore safely. From shoulder to shoulder and hip to hip, your torso creates a "box" or square that serves as a reference for the rest of your body (*opposite*). To avoid unnecessary twisting, always work with a square box, imagining yourself from all angles. During each exercise, ask yourself: "Am I square?" It is not uncommon to favour one side of the body. You may find yourself consistently leaning or rotating to one side. Train your eyes to detect and adjust any misalignments you see.

THE POWERHOUSE

The powerhouse is simply a label that Pilates teachers use to describe the collective muscles of your abdominals, gluteals (buttock muscles), and lower back musculature. We define the powerhouse as the centre of strength and control for the rest of your body. Pilates practitioners also

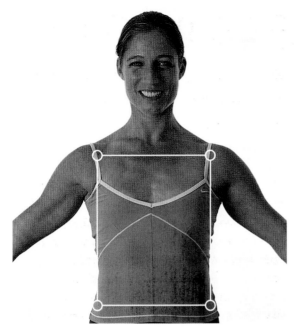

The Box The four lines connecting shoulder to shoulder, shoulders to hips, and hip to hip create a perfect square or "box". This visual representation serves as a continuous reminder of symmetry as you work.

refer to this region as your "girdle of strength" or your "core muscles". Many of us exercise without paying attention to the initiation or beginning of each movement. As a result, we move improperly and suffer a series of strains, pulls, and injuries. Pilates will train you to recruit your powerhouse as you begin every movement.

"The less the average person merely talks about health, the better it is for his health."

In each exercise you perform, you will be instructed to begin by activating and engaging your powerhouse before all other muscle groups. In this way you will learn to initiate each exercise from the centre of your body. This technique will strengthen and protect your body for a lifetime.

GLOSSARY

Below are the most common terms used in Pilates, with a brief definition of what each phrase means.

Alignment The position or place where the joints of the body are both in line and symmetrical.

Articulate the Spine The movement of the spine so that each segment is clearly distinguished or differentiated from the next as you move through the spinal column.

Box The area defined from shoulder to shoulder and hip to hip, which serves as a self-reference for your alignment.

Chin to Chest The position assumed when the body is supine and the head is lifted. The weight of the head is drawn towards the chest, without resulting tension.

Dynamics The motion of a body part as a result of the energy you perform it with. Dynamics are unique to each exercise.

Navel to Spine; Scoop The drawing inwards and upwards of the abdominal muscles and particularly the transverse abdominals, resulting in a hollow or scooped appearance in the waistline.

Opposition The act of using a muscle group or body part in an opposing way to another muscle group or body part.

Pilates Stance or Position The tensing of the gluteal or buttock muscles to effect the rotating or wrapping of the legs together from the hips to the heels, resulting in a tripod position with the feet.

Powerhouse; Girdle of Strength; Core Muscles The band of muscles encircling the torso and extending from the lower rib cage to just below the buttocks.

Stabilize; Anchor; Plant The activation or engagement of the core muscles to fix the body in a position from which it is not easily adjusted.

Threshold The level of work where you are only just able to complete the activity. In exercise, we strive to work our muscles at threshold. Working below threshold will greatly reduce the benefit to your muscles.

Wings Down The act of sliding or depressing the shoulder blades down the back and away from the neck and head.

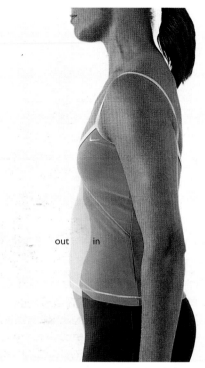

out   in

"Scoop" Here the action of the abdominal muscles pulling backwards towards the spine is illustrated. Note that the upper body does not round forwards to effect the action of scooping. Nor do the hips shift forwards. The scoop is purely muscular and the skeleton should not move.

THE ACT OF SCOOPING

One afternoon during the photo shoot of this book, the photographer steadied his camera, focused on the model, and yelled "Scoop". Having listened to me coach the models for several days, he had internalized the concept without ever trying to perform a Pilates exercise.

Perhaps more than any other concept in this book, you will read the words "navel to spine" or "scoop the abdominals in and up". Even the finest of athletes have difficulty with this concept. Your abdominals run lengthwise in the case of the rectus abdominis (your "six-pack") and diagonally in the case of your "obliques" (or waistline muscles). The Pilates technique is primarily concerned with the lateral band of muscles known as the transverse abdominals. This muscle encircles the waistline

from front to back and, when contracted, pulls the abdominal wall inwards towards the spine, decreasing the dimension of your waist. In fact, the actual muscle fibres of the transverse surround your six-pack muscles, pulling the rectus inwards each time the transverse is contracted.

Imagine the abdominal wall as a moving walkway at an airport that moves from your belly button to your backbone. The act of "scooping" involves moving this muscular walkway directly through the body from front to back. You may also compare the sensation of pulling the navel to the spine to the tightening of a corset around your waist or the pulling in required to zip up a tight pair of trousers. So long as the distance between the navel and the spine decreases, it doesn't matter what image you use. What is important is that you do not change the alignment of your bones in order to contract your muscles. In other words, do not shorten the waist, round the shoulders forwards, or thrust the hips under just to pull your waistline in. The activity is restricted solely to the abdominal muscles.

CONTROLLED MOBILITY

Infants are born with too many neurons (also known as nerve endings). Arms and legs move wildly in seemingly random patterns. Over time, neurons find other neurons and build pathways to create specific movement patterns. These developmental pathways are dictated by desire and will. If a child wants to grasp a toy, he must rehearse the task repeatedly. Ultimately, he is able to perform the desired movement. This pattern always begins at the centre of the body and works its way to the periphery. Once the body core is stable, the limbs have a greater degree of controlled mobility. For example, if your shoulder is moving around, you cannot possibly place your hand in a particular spot. Your entire Pilates workout will address the strength and control of your torso, thereby freeing the limbs to move without risk of injury. As you develop your core strength, you will learn to move from a stable base with maximum control.

OPENING THE CHEST

To enhance posture, restore alignment, and improve breathing, the action of opening the chest cannot be understated. Be careful not to over-expand the ribs, which will cause them to thrust forwards of your hips. Your spinal alignment should be preserved at all times. Imagine yourself assuming a military posture: the head is high, the chest is lifted, and the shoulders are held back and down.

ACTIVATING THE WINGS

For many of us, the neck and shoulders store tension. When the body experiences effort or strain, the muscles in this area automatically react and seize up. Rather than allow this involuntary response, we can use these muscles to assist us as we exercise.

> "The mistreated body, mindful of its past neglect, eventually exacts repayment in full with interest."

Your shoulder blades rest outside of your rib cage without any bony attachment to the spine. Shrug your shoulders several times and you will feel how they glide easily up and down your back. The act of "pulling the wings down" involves actively pressing the shoulder blades lower than their normal resting position. This motion of depressing the shoulders or sliding them down and back will simultaneously lengthen the neck, strengthen the back, and eliminate neck and shoulder tension.

OPPOSITION

For every action there is an equal and opposite reaction. As you work out, you will be using opposition to balance, counterbalance, and stabilize your body. Picture yourself on a merry-go-round reaching from your horse for the brass ring in the centre. To sustain a position, one side of your body reaches away as the other side opposes your

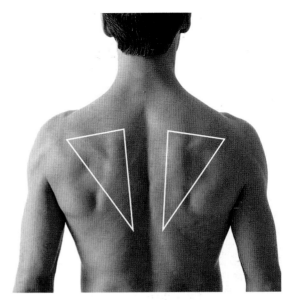

"Wings Down" The shoulder blades are two, free-floating triangles that migrate downwards and inwards towards the spine. Continue to open the chest as you press the wings down and back. In exercises where you are reclined, imagine the front of your shoulders pinned back to the mat

reach. Without this natural opposition, your balance would be compromised and you would simply fall off your horse. In Pilates, we train our bodies to emphasize these opposing motions, thereby increasing our control and stabilization and ultimately our strength.

DYNAMICS

Movement energies are specific. Each exercise has changing dynamics just as music compositions have a prelude, a peak, and a conclusion. As you progress through the workout, pay attention to words like "emphasize" or "accent" and perform this part with a little extra vigour. Dynamics lend each exercise rhythm and quality as well as dictate which part should speed up or slow down. Controlling the tempo of a movement ensures that you receive the most intense possible challenge from each exercise. Be careful not to confuse dynamics with momentum. Words like "upswing" do not imply that you should move so forcefully so as to sacrifice

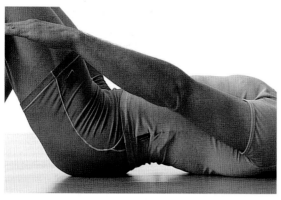

Do not arch your back or allow a large space between the floor and your spine to occur. This places stress on the lower back and makes it difficult to recruit the powerhouse.

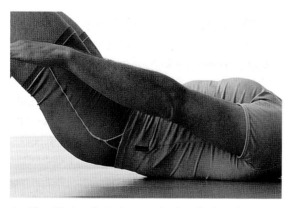

Avoid tucking or flattening your back so far into the mat that the hips lift off the floor. This serves only to over-contract the hip sockets and grip the surrounding muscles.

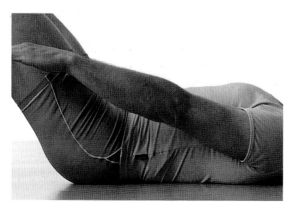

A correctly aligned spine, neither tucked nor arched but lengthened, allows the best recruitment of core musculature.

your form. Each exercise requires the perfect balance of energy and control. Lastly, incorporating the appropriate dynamic of each exercise requires the use of your breath and will help to improve the flow of your workout.

NEUTRAL SPINE

There is much talk of neutral spine in the Pilates world today. This concept had no bearing on Mr Pilates' original technique, but it will help to illuminate the use of your spine as you navigate your way in and out of this book.

The phrase "neutral spine" defines the place where your spine rests while preserving all of its natural curves. This is easily accomplished while standing upright but, when gravity is a factor, as it is when lying down, the correct alignment of your spine may be harder to establish.

Avoiding Common Pitfalls

There are two common pitfalls to avoid. The first is known as "tucking under". It defines the motion of tilting the hips so that the lower part of the pelvis rises up and the upper part tips down or back. Many Pilates exercises direct you to keep your back flat on the mat, but you do not want to flatten so much that the buttocks rise up or the hip muscles grip. When standing or sitting, tucking under can also have the undesirable effect of flattening the natural curve of the lumbar (lower) spine.

The opposite of tucking under occurs when the abdominal muscles are not yet strong enough to sustain a position and the lower back muscles contract into an arched position, allowing the stomach muscles to protrude. Both of these conditions can be hazardous and neither is correct. For proper alignment, simply lengthen your spine along the mat and concentrate on isolating your abdominal scoop without shifting your pelvis.

Maintaining a Strong Body

Pilates was developed with the idea that people spend most of their working day in poor postural alignment. Prolonged sitting coupled with improper body mechanics make it impossible for the spine to receive a balanced

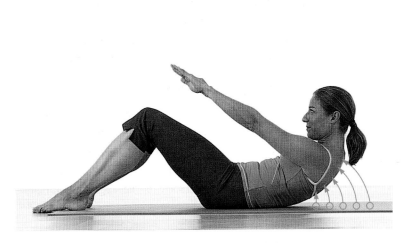

Spinal Articulation The spine works segment by segment, rolling up and down through the floor and articulating each section. In this photograph, as the model rises up off the mat, her spine curves, increasing the distance between her and the floor. The same action will result as she reverses the motion, lowering her spine to the mat one vertebra at a time. The goal is a strong but mobile spine.

diet of movement. The original programme called for a solid mixture of spinal flexion (bending forwards) and extension (bending backwards) exercises, providing a total workout for the spine. As people began to approach Pilates as a rehabilitative technique, many of the extension exercises were reserved for advanced students with healthy spines. Thus the Pilates programme became largely a flexion programme. Here, in *Pilates: Body in Motion,* I have presented the full matwork programme. Bear in mind that these exercises were created for the healthy individual. In theory and in practice, this complete workout addresses the entire body and will help you to maintain a strong body and a healthy back.

SPINAL ARTICULATION

There are several expressions used throughout this book to convey the mobility of the spine. Wherever you read "articulate the spine" or "curl the spine vertebra by vertebra", your goal is to work through each part of the spine, mobilizing and separating each vertebra. As you curl and uncurl your spine, you will feel sections that resist mobility. These stiff spots are the areas where you must linger and breathe to increase the opening of the area. Whether you are rising or lowering, concentrate on actively configuring your spine into a "C" shape in order to increase mobility and strength.

WORKING AT THRESHOLD

Each of us possesses a unique tolerance level with respect to our physical ability. To increase your level of proficiency, you must increase this tolerance or threshold, whether it be your strength, flexibility, or endurance. Each exercise should be performed at the point where you can only just complete the exercise while still adhering to all the instructions. If, while performing a push up, you can barely bend and straighten your arms, you are already at threshold. Practise this exercise until you can bend the arms a bit more and ultimately even further. If, on the other hand, you are able to lower your body down and up with ease, you will need to find the aspects of the exercise that are difficult for you. Perhaps it is maintaining your spine and head in one line, perhaps you need to place your arms more correctly, or your legs. Understanding that there is always a way to work harder in any given exercise will help you truly become your own teacher.

THE USE OF IMAGERY

Images are tools to help you catch the essence of a movement and are key to the Pilates method. Imagery can be as simple as pretending your entire body is something else, or it can be more specific to a certain body part. The more complex images are those that require you to move with certain characteristics. For example, you may read the

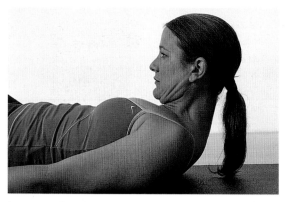

Improper placement, with the chin held too close to the chest, causes muscle tension in the jaw as well as shortening of the muscles of the neck.

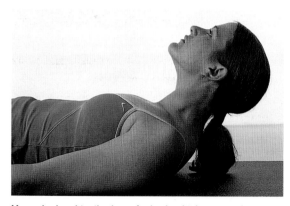

Here, the head is tilted too far back, which can result in strain to the muscles in the front of the neck as well as bulging of the abdominal wall.

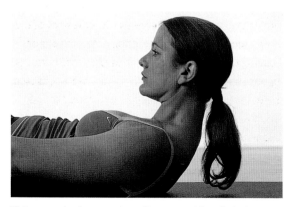

This example shows correct alignment, with a slight space under the chin and the eyes focused toward the midsection.

following: "Roll your spine down to the mat just like dripping honey." Here the image of honey is meant to convey that the movement is slow and smooth. Imagery is just another way to improve your precision and drive your concentration. In order to use imagery effectively, you must establish your own internal dialogue or inner voice. Train yourself to coach your body through each movement, dictating mentally the motions and images for each segment of every exercise.

CHIN TO CHEST

In exercises that call for the body to remain flat on the floor with the head and limbs elevated, the position of the head is vital. Other exercise techniques use the image of an egg or some other object placed under the chin during abdominal exercises. In Pilates we use the weight of the head drawn forwards to help decrease neck tension and thereby increase the work of the abdominals.

Bringing the chin too far down, where it presses against the neck, is incorrect and uncomfortable. Conversely, leaving the head behind you will strain the front of the neck muscles and make it difficult to maintain correct spinal alignment. The correct alignment places the head above the sternum (breastbone) with a space underneath the chin and the eyes focused on the midsection or girdle area. This position also facilitates the best possible recruitment of the powerhouse.

A SAFE "FRAME"

The word "frame" is sometimes used interchangeably with the word "box" (*see p15*), but it has a different meaning and should be treated as a distinct concept. To work within your frame means to keep your limbs in control and within the scope of your box, or torso. Though Pilates aims to increase flexibility of overly tight areas, we do not stretch beyond neutral or seek to increase a joint's range of motion beyond its normal functional limits. We are not concerned with achieving high-kicking legs or the splits of a gymnast, but only with the optimal motion of the body. For example, in the beginner's programme you will

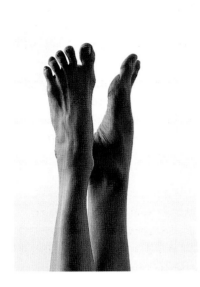

Pilates position is demonstrated here in two ways. With the legs in the air (*left*), the position is established by wrapping or rotating the backs of the legs and buttocks together. The feet respond by opening into a tripod position. In standing (*right*), the effect is the same. By activating the buttocks and legs the feet will assume the shape of a small letter "V".

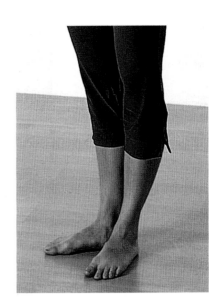

perform a series of circular arm movements as you lean against a wall. You will be directed to keep the arms moving within the peripheral vision. Although the arms travel wider than your torso, they never go beyond the line of the joint, whether it be overhead or out to the side. Each Pilates exercise keeps your limbs working in a safe range.

LENGTHENING

A dear friend of mine went to a dance audition when she was just 11 years old. She was eliminated immediately because she was too short for the part. Waiting outside was her dance teacher who, upon hearing this, told the young dancer, "Go back in ... and be the right height!" She did, and she was, and she got the part.

Pilates teachers speak often of lifting and lengthening, growing higher and pulling up taller. Is this really possible? How can one simply be taller? As you read the directives "Stretch up tall" and "Lengthen out", you should focus on creating distance between the hipbones and the rib cage, which will have the effect of elongating your waist. Anatomically speaking, this motion actually lengthens your spine and decompresses your vertebrae. Improving your posture in this way can temporarily give you the appearance of more height. Strengthening and

reeducating your postural muscles to sustain this posture will improve your stature forever.

As you work to lengthen your limbs, be certain that you do not lock or jam your joints. Work your muscles but not your bones. Do not hyperextend your arms or legs, straightening them past normal or neutral alignment, as this can weaken your muscles.

PILATES STANCE

Pilates stance is commonly described as a foot position. The heels come together and the toes open slightly, placing the feet in a "V" shape. However, Pilates stance is not defined by the shape of the feet. It is the work of the powerhouse that initiates the action of turning out or rotating the legs. By squeezing or wrapping the buttocks tightly and pressing the backs of the thighs towards each other, the legs respond by rotating into a small tripod position. It is critical to remember the phrase "work from the knee up, not the knee down" when establishing this position. The muscular action occurs in the core of the body and not in the periphery. Pilates stance performed while lying down is no different. The feet and lower legs maintain a long, loose, relaxed position, while the buttocks and inner thighs are activated.

LEARNING PILATES

What is the most effective means of learning this method? Obviously, your grasp of this system depends upon your baseline level of fitness and your ability to translate words and pictures into movements. There are, however, several elements that are necessary and invaluable to the absorption of Pilates.

Memorization

Memorization is required. You will need to retain mentally each exercise in your routine. This will drive you to improve your programme rather than just get through it. Start with the beginner workout and practise listing the exercises in the order that they are performed. Once you can rattle off the titles of each exercise, you can then focus on connecting and flowing your programme together with the use of transitions.

Transitions

Each exercise in the series is linked to the next by way of a specific transition. As you advance your workout, begin to incorporate these movements. The transitions in the Pilates programme are choreographed to keep your body engrossed in the workout. The human body does whatever is necessary to avoid muscular exertion and the lapse between movements is the obvious place to rest. Transitions thus become very important. They remind you not to rest. In linking exercises together, you will begin to learn by flow. You will find yourself stringing exercises together without thinking about what comes next. Each transition uses a minimum of movement to conserve energy and help speed your workout. In this way both your endurance and your vascular capacity are enhanced.

Quality and Tempo

Once your technique has developed and you have a grasp of the order of the series, the next element is quality. Imagine yourself performing the exercises before a live audience. When technical prowess exceeds a certain level, the work becomes effortless. As you become more proficient in Pilates, your muscles should glide easily in and out of shapes, flowing easily without any locking of your joints or unnecessary tension.

As your workout advances, so too should your speed or tempo. The transitions between exercises will begin to flow together, but so should the movements within exercises. Ideally, the matwork becomes one seamless movement from the first exercise to the last. Mr Pilates said that his method should be performed at the rhythm of your heart. Keep your tempo brisk and even, but do not sacrifice the quality of your movement for speed.

> "The benefits of Pilates depend solely on your performing the exercises exactly according to the instructions."

Advancing your workout by rushing your progress and adding new material is very tempting but will not accurately reflect your progress. Pilates cannot be measured by how many exercises you know or how many repetitions you can perform. Your mastery of the method occurs in layers, beginning with your understanding of the mechanics of the movement and ending with the integration of your body and mind.

The inherent design of Pilates ensures that its benefits will transfer to your real life and the physical gains you achieve in your workout will be reflected in your everyday activities. You need only get started.

MOTIVATION

So you have a mat and you've got the book and you are ready. How do you get into the mood to exercise? What will be your motivation?

Your first strategy will be to change how you think about exercise. Once you are practising Pilates regularly, you will automatically change the way you think about fitness but, in the beginning, you may need to modify your approach. Begin by simply changing the label. Don't say, "I'm going to work out now." Instead say, "I'm going to do Pilates." Pilates is work — but it is gratifying work that will energize and rejuvenate you. Next, imagine your routine as a luxury event, like a long bath or a massage. The opportunity to mentally escape from your external life and focus on your internal wellbeing is a wonderful respite from your daily routine. Finally, as you lower to the mat, think to yourself, "I'm just going to lie down, stretch out for a minute, take a few deep breaths and say hello to my body." Then do just that. Lengthen out along your mat, breathe deeply, and begin with the first exercise. It is perfectly fine if you stop there. You may only perform one exercise the first couple of times. Soon after you will add the next exercise. What is most important is that you introduce regular movement into your everyday routine.

The Benefit of Regular Practice

In his original book *Return to Life through Contrology*, Mr Pilates suggested you begin with just 10 minutes every day. His suggestion was well founded. With regular practice, your body will begin to change from the inside out. With only 10 minutes a day, you will begin to feel the effects of this method. You may not be aware of them at first, but you will notice that when you skip a day you feel differently. By the time you feel ready to expand your routine, you will have a whole new perspective on exercise and a keen appreciation of what your body is capable of.

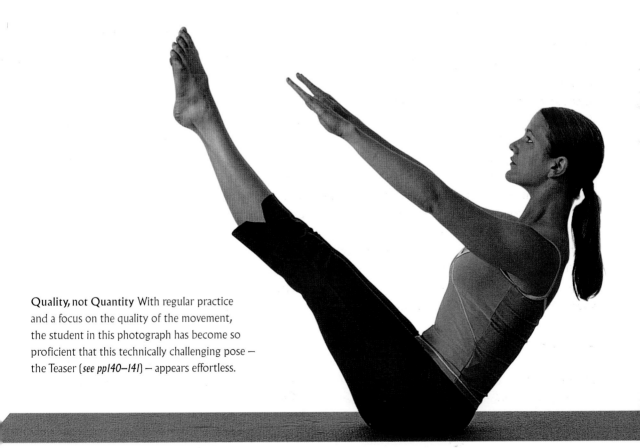

Quality, not Quantity With regular practice and a focus on the quality of the movement, the student in this photograph has become so proficient that this technically challenging pose — the Teaser (*see pp140–141*) — appears effortless.

BEGINNING PILATES

There is no right way or perfect time to begin your study of the Pilates method. There are, however, a number of guidelines that will help you to optimize the benefits and to enhance your experience.

• Dress comfortably. Ideally you should wear clothes that make it easy to see the shapes that your body is making. Either socks or bare feet are appropriate.

• Do not eat within the hour preceding your workout.

• Use a mat to protect your spine. If a mat is not available, use blankets or large towels to create a cushioned surface.

• Practise often. It is best if you invest a lot of your time as you are learning the material and then taper off once you have a solid routine. Pilates can be done every day.

• Perform only the basic introductory and/or beginner routine for the first 4–6 weeks, then add one new exercise at a time from the intermediate workout. Before trying any advanced material, you should be able to complete the full intermediate programme in under 30 minutes.

HOW TO USE THIS BOOK

The exercise section of the book includes several visual elements to guide you through your workout.

Colour Each level is colour-coded to help you distinguish which section you are in, from introductory and

beginner's programmes to intermediate and advanced. Each level is treated separately, but your work builds on a mastery of the exercises in the preceding chapter.

Cue boxes at the beginning of each movement direct you through the number of repetitions suggested as well as contraindications and helpful visualization tools.

Head–to–Toe Checklists are included with most exercises, providing pointers and tips to help improve your form. Remind yourself of these corrections throughout the exercise. The accompanying photographs demonstrate the most commonly made mistakes. The contrast between right and wrong should be glaringly obvious.

Modifications Many exercises include modified versions. Examine these to see if they apply to you before attempting the traditional version. This book contains four levels of workouts and numerous modifications, which should address most physical limitations.

At a Glance Each exercise is laid out in a miniature exercise sequence at the bottom of the page to remind you of the breathing that accompanies each movement. Refer to these sequences to prompt you through your workout.

Transitions are provided for each exercise. Where appropriate, I have given you the option of segueing into either the advanced or the intermediate exercise. With the

No Equipment Required The matwork is the most accessible part of the Pilates method and requires no equipment other than a mat or padded surface to protect the delicate vertebrae of your spine. Find an area that is large enough to accommodate the entire length of your body with your

arms extended overhead and your legs stretched out to their fullest. There is no special attire or footwear required. You need only dress comfortably in clothing that allows you to move easily and to supervise your form. Lie flat on your back to begin your workout.

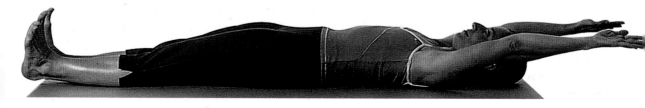

exception of the introductory workout, which contains its own transitions, the remaining levels all connect in the traditional, advanced order.

Sequence Charts demonstrate the correct order of exercises in the intermediate and advanced sections (beginner workouts stand alone). Once you have learned the exercises individually, try working out using only the chart. Never skip around the book: if you are unsure of the order, refer back to the sequence charts.

MODIFICATION NOTES

Mr Pilates created his method for the "normal, healthy body". The nature of each injury is unique and should never be self-diagnosed. Above all, never work through pain. Every exercise should be performed in a pain-free range. To keep your body safe but still working at threshold, you will need to distinguish between effort and strain. The effort of hard work is appropriate, but strain can cause damage. A sharp pain anywhere is always a warning sign and should be attended to immediately.

Working with Injuries

For weak or injured necks If holding your head up while lying flat causes you pain, simply leave it down. If possible, lift it for brief periods and rest intermittently. Avoid exercises that require you to roll onto your neck. For some, a rolled towel or cushion under the head may provide relief.

Shoulders, Elbows, or Wrists Injuries to the upper limbs may prohibit certain weight-bearing exercises. For shoulder injuries, pay attention to your range of motion, working slowly and carefully in a shortened range.

Backs Back injuries demand that you proceed with caution. Exercises where you remain flat on your back or your stomach are considered to be the safest. Delay adding exercises that involve rolling or twisting the spine. If you have no history of back pain, but are experiencing a diffuse ache in the "girdle area" or a dull pain that surrounds the waistline and dissipates as the exercise concludes, you may simply be suffering from muscle fatigue as your transverse abdominals gain strength.

Nonetheless, remember never to work through pain.

Hips If you experience hip pain while one or both legs are moving in the air, try softening or slightly bending your knees. Hip injuries may also restrict the degree of forward bending you can perform. These movements should be performed slowly and carefully within a pain-free range.

Knees and Ankles A knee or ankle injury may limit your ability to kneel or completely straighten your leg. Pay attention to the symmetry and alignment of your legs as you work out. Avoid hyperextending your knees as well as bending them in too tightly, both of which can aggravate an existing injury.

Static Stretching

Stretching can cause injury when performed improperly. To increase flexibility you must perform what is known as "static stretching". Do not bounce your body while in a stretched position, as this has the opposite effect, and will serve only to tighten your muscles. Instead, breathe deeply and relax into the stretch with each breath.

Remember, also, that a condition that requires you to adjust an exercise should never discourage you. Pilates is uniquely adaptable and just about everyone can do it.

A WORD ABOUT PREGNANCY

There has been a growing trend for women to explore Pilates as an exercise option during the early or middle stages of pregnancy. New exercise regimes are generally discouraged during pregnancy and the extreme focus on the abdominal wall makes Pilates an unlikely choice for a pregnant woman with no prior experience. However, if you are a Pilates veteran and are already familiar with the exercises in this book, or if you are currently working out with a teacher, you may continue your visits, but with a modified routine. Ask your instructor to choose which exercises would be appropriate for you at your level. Finally, for a post-partum routine, Pilates is ideal. Begin immediately after your doctor has given you clearance. Take your time, work deeply and carefully, and results will be rapidly yours.

PREPARATION EXERCISE

In this exercise, which serves as a welcome mat, you will begin to integrate the principles you have just been reading about. In many instances, the Preparation exercise also provides a transition from one exercise to another. Begin slowly, with focus and concentration, allowing no part of your body to escape your control.

REPETITIONS Once only.

CAUTION If you find that you are unable to rise up without distending the abdominals, use the modified version (see p28).

VISUALIZATION Imagine slowly peeling your spine off the mat from top to bottom, just as you would peel a piece of tape off something delicate.

glue legs
tightly
together

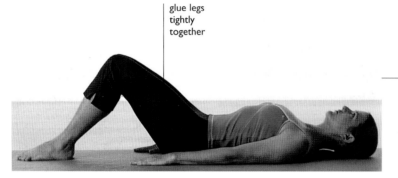

1 Lie on your back with knees bent and arms long on the mat. Take three deep breaths. With each breath feel your navel sinking down closer to your backbone.

2 Initiating from your powerhouse (*see p14*), inhale and lift your head and shoulders up, reaching your arms to the opposite end of the room. Keep your eyes on your waistline. Do not let the abdominals protrude: instead, breathe laterally (*see p14*).

arms reach
out long

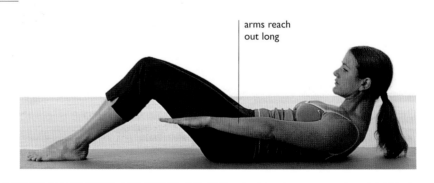

At a glance

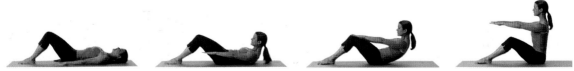

Inhale to begin.......................Exhale to roll up...................................Rest

3 As you exhale, peel the spine up off the mat, articulating each spinal segment, vertebra by vertebra (*see p19*). The feet should remain firmly planted on the floor, with the knees bent at a 90° angle and legs pressed firmly together.

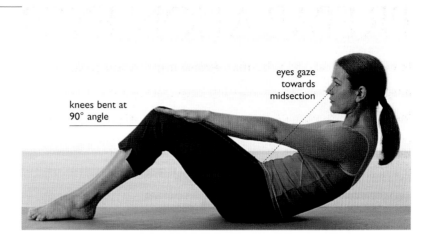

knees bent at 90° angle

eyes gaze towards midsection

4 Finish by sitting up tall. Scoop the abdominals in and up (*see p16*) and continue to press the legs tightly together. TRANSITION: *Roll slowly back down to the mat and bring the knees in to the chest to prepare for the Introductory Hundred* (see pp32–33).

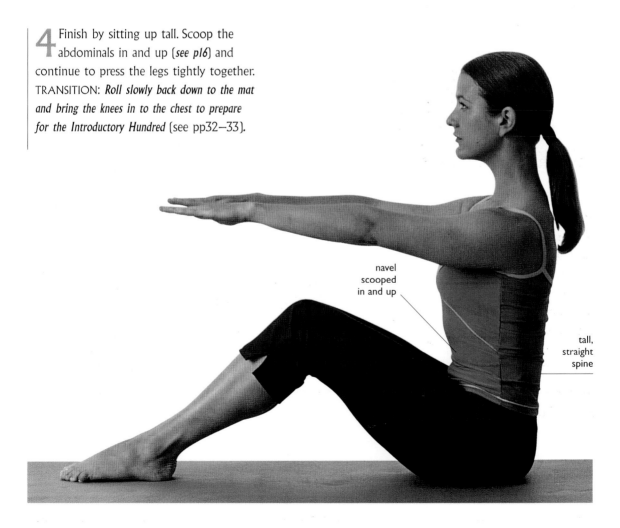

navel scooped in and up

tall, straight spine

MODIFIED HAND POSITION
You may use your hands to assist you in curling up.
Keep the elbows wide and press the "wings" (*see p17*)
down, sliding the shoulder blades down the back.
Continue to sink the waist deeper as you rise up.

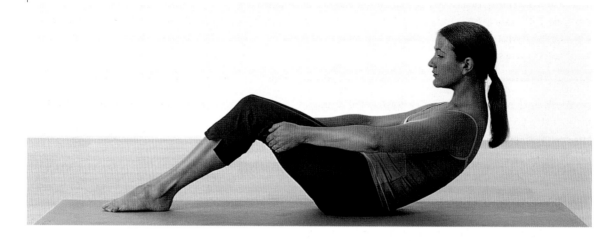

HEAD-TO-TOE CHECKLIST

• **Draw** the weight of the head forward as you bring your chin to your chest (*see p20*). You may place your neck at risk if you leave your head behind you when curling up.

• **Slowly curl up** using the resistance of the floor to articulate your spine.

Bringing your body up too quickly can cause you to lose your abdominal power and the C-curve (*see p19*) in your back.

• **Keep** your feet anchored to the floor and your inner thighs drawn together throughout the sequence.

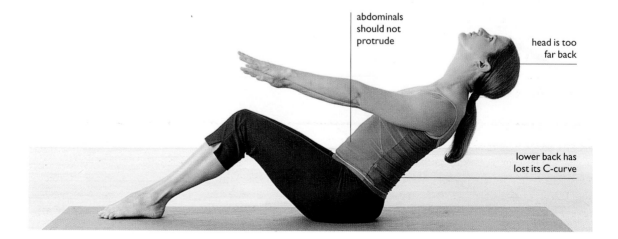

abdominals
should not
protrude

head is too
far back

lower back has
lost its C-curve

SELF-EVALUATION

The Preparation exercise was designed to make you aware of the numerous concepts required to perform successfully one simple movement. In order to negotiate this system and see the results of your work, you must actively think your way through each movement. Let's analyze the exercise. Basically you took a few breaths and then sat up. Right? Well, yes ... but is that really all that happened? Ask yourself the following questions:

Was it hard? If it wasn't, something is wrong. Try the exercise again, more slowly and thoughtfully this time. Then ask yourself why it was hard. What specifically was difficult? Was it the movement? Was it the positioning? Was it the breath? Or was it the fact that there were so many details?

The details are the essence of Pilates. The details are what separate this method from all other forms of exercise. The details and your attention to them will change your body. Let's examine the details of the Preparation exercise.

- [ ] The neck is long on the mat as you lie flat
- [ ] When lying flat, the legs are together
- [ ] The knees are bent at a 90° angle throughout
- [ ] The navel is pulled in to the spine
- [ ] As you roll up, the arms reach forwards just off the mat
- [ ] The feet cannot move as you roll up
- [ ] The spine must articulate smoothly, vertebra by vertebra
- [ ] The abdominals must pull in tightly as you come up to sit tall

What about the details of the method that were not mentioned but are always present?

- [ ] Were you symmetrical?
- [ ] Did you keep your box square?
- [ ] Were you working your transverse abdominals to scoop your navel to your spine?
- [ ] Were you working your wings to pull your shoulders down and keep your neck relaxed?
- [ ] Was the movement controlled?
- [ ] Was it fluid?
- [ ] Was it precise?

Finally ... were you concentrating? It is my wish to bring the instructor to you; in the absence of that possibility I must empower you to become your own instructor. If you continue with this system of self-evaluation throughout each and every exercise, you will have truly mastered the science of learning Pilates. Your physical ability can always be improved upon, but realizing your fullest potential depends upon your ability to coach yourself. Use this book to become your own teacher. Learn how to pinpoint each mistake. Then ask yourself, "How can I correct it and make it better?" In this way, your practice of Pilates will continue to improve and to inspire you for a lifetime. Good Luck and Enjoy!

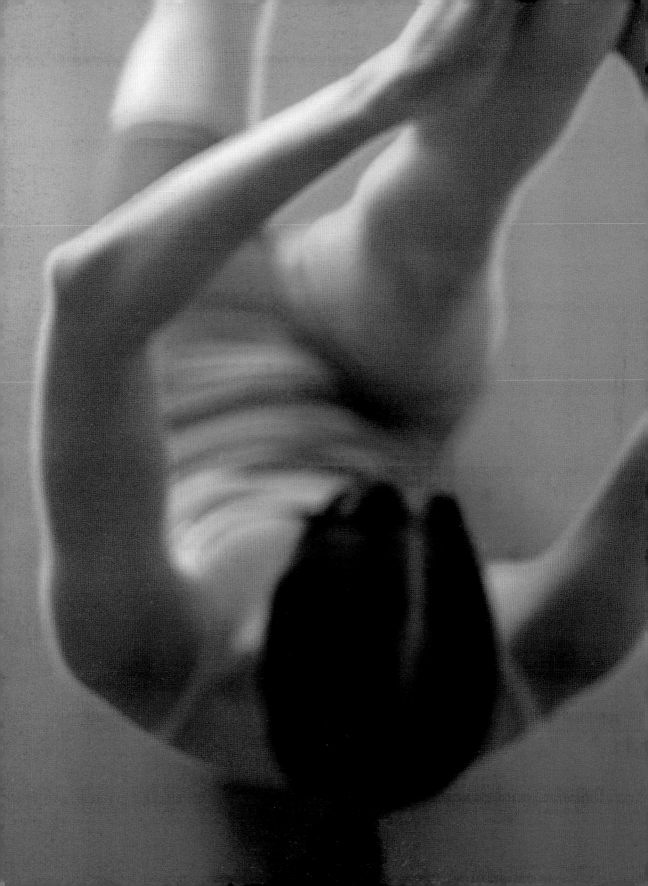

1

INTRODUCTORY PROGRAMME

The Introductory Programme is designed to integrate the Pilates exercises with their corresponding ideals and concepts. Here, the Pilates principles of *breath* and *concentration* are developed, establishing a foundation for the entire system. Try to perform this routine daily, even if only for ten minutes.

THE HUNDRED

The Hundred is the first exercise of Joseph Pilates' original regimen. In this introductory version, you will warm up your body to prepare for the rest of the matwork. Inhale fully and exhale completely throughout the exercise – these deep breaths will stimulate your circulation and build stamina.

REPETITIONS 5–10 sets of full breath cycles (50–100 pumps).

CAUTION A shoulder injury may limit your ability to pump your arms. You may simply reach long, or pump softly. If you develop neck pain, lower your head.

VISUALIZATION Imagine your lungs are like balloons that expand and collapse with each breath.

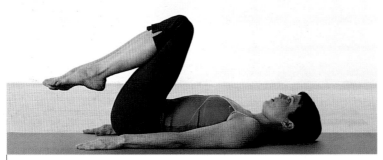

1 Lie on your back to begin, with both knees drawn in to the chest. Feel the entire length of your spine on the mat.

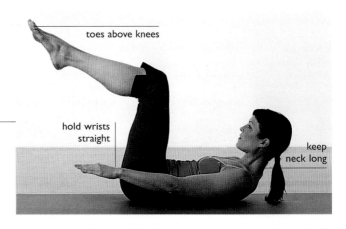

toes above knees

hold wrists straight

keep neck long

2 Use your powerhouse to lift your head and shoulders up, reaching the arms just above the mat. Extend your legs up, keeping your knees bent and the toes just above the knees.

At a glance

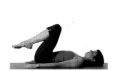 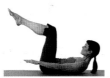 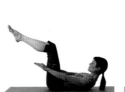 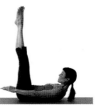 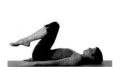

Breathe in for 5 pumps.................Breathe out for 5 pumps......................Rest

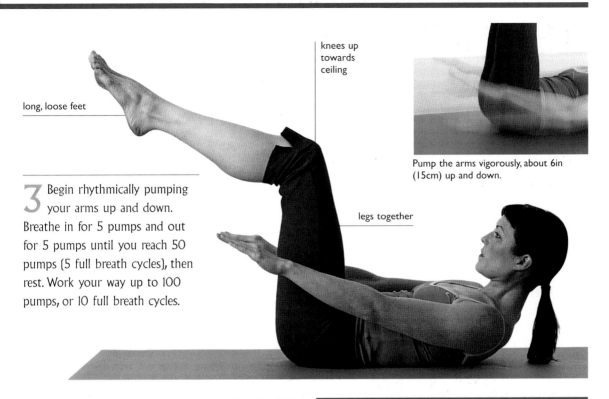

long, loose feet

knees up towards ceiling

Pump the arms vigorously, about 6in (15cm) up and down.

legs together

3 Begin rhythmically pumping your arms up and down. Breathe in for 5 pumps and out for 5 pumps until you reach 50 pumps (5 full breath cycles), then rest. Work your way up to 100 pumps, or 10 full breath cycles.

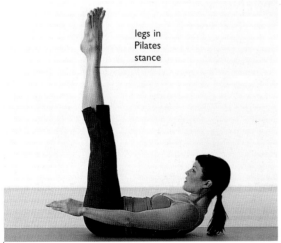

legs in Pilates stance

4 To increase the difficulty of the exercise, you may straighten both legs up to the ceiling. When finished, lower your head and draw the knees in to the chest, returning to Step 1 position.
TRANSITION: *Place both feet on the mat to prepare for the Roll Down (see pp34–35).*

HEAD-TO-TOE CHECKLIST

- **Do not** bend the wrists while pumping. Keep stretching through the fingertips.
- **Keep arms** synchronized while pumping.
- **Do not allow** the knees to sink towards the chest.
- **The toes** remain above the knees and the knees aim directly for the ceiling.
- **Avoid** shallow breathing: inhale fully and exhale completely.

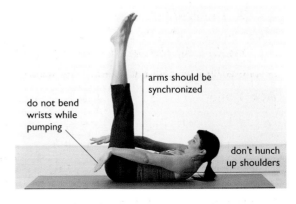

do not bend wrists while pumping

arms should be synchronized

don't hunch up shoulders

ROLL DOWN

The Roll Down is an essential precursor to many of our rolling exercises. Focus on actively scooping in your navel – as you work the abdominals towards the spine you should see your midsection hollowing out. The awareness and control you develop in this exercise will be your foundation for the rest of the matwork.

> **REPETITIONS** Repeat entire sequence 3 times.
>
> **CAUTION** Hold the legs lightly if you have a wrist, elbow, or shoulder impairment.
>
> **VISUALIZATION** Imagine your hipbones and lower ribs as large dots on your torso: try to "connect the dots" with each exhalation, sinking the abdominals deeper.

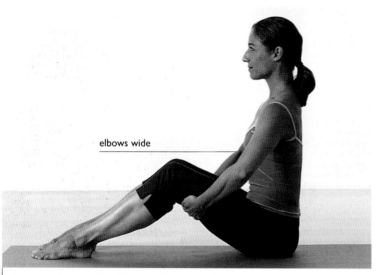

elbows wide

1 Begin sitting tall with your heels on the mat and your feet as flat as possible. The legs are parallel and hip width apart. Wrap the hands behind the thighs and lift the elbows wide. Draw the waistline in and up.

2 Engage your buttocks and curl your pelvis under you, aiming your lower back towards the floor. Simultaneously tilt your chin down and look into your midsection, shaping your spine into a C-curve (*see p19*).

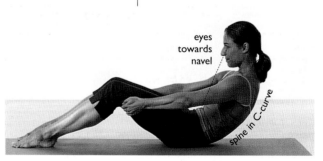

eyes towards navel

spine in C-curve

At a glance

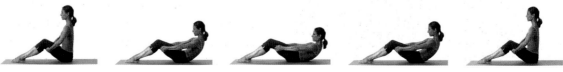

Breathe naturally..................Breathe in and out 3 times......................Repeat

3 Increase the C-curve, pressing your spine firmly into the mat. Hold this position and take 3 deep breaths, opening the muscles of the lower back as the abdominals pull in deeper. Curl back up to your starting position, sinking the waist in even deeper. Repeat 3 times.
TRANSITION: *Lower down to the mat with your arms by your sides and your knees bent for the Single Leg Circles* (see pp36–37).

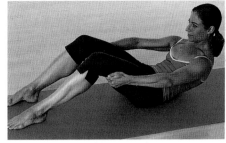

Keep the legs hip width apart and in proper alignment as you curl back up.

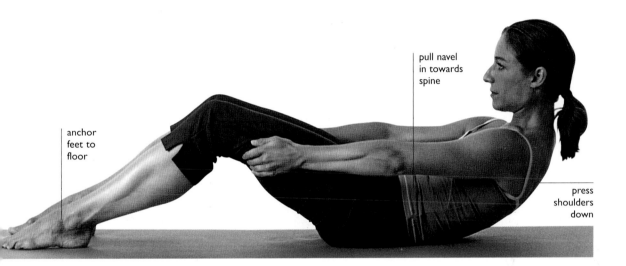

anchor feet to floor

pull navel in towards spine

press shoulders down

HEAD-TO-TOE CHECKLIST

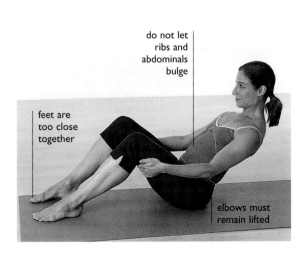

do not let ribs and abdominals bulge

feet are too close together

elbows must remain lifted

• **Avoid** leaning the upper body back. Initiate the movement from the base of the spine rather than from the upper back.
• **Do not allow** the rib cage and abdominals to project outwards – this encourages your lower back to arch and places you at risk of injury.
• **Ensure that your** elbows remain lifted.

• **Work slowly** and concentrate on bringing the belly button towards the backbone.
• **Keep** the feet fixed on the mat with the knees at a 90° angle. Bringing them in towards the buttocks increases the difficulty.
• **If your toes** do not touch the mat with your knees at a right angle, keep the heels on the mat.

SINGLE LEG CIRCLES

This leg circling exercise will strengthen your hip muscles while increasing flexibility. Use the exercise to work on pulling your "wings" down without sacrificing your powerhouse. Throughout the movement, anchor your body to the mat and use your leg like a paintbrush tracing perfect circles in the air.

REPETITIONS 5 times in each direction, clockwise and anti-clockwise, with each leg.

CAUTION If you feel any strain in the back of the knee, you may slightly soften the knee.

VISUALIZATION Visualize your leg as a long, slender paintbrush tracing circles in the air.

Start the exercise with your navel drawn in and up.

1 Lie flat on the mat with your neck long and your right leg up to the ceiling. The left knee is bent and the left foot is firmly planted on the mat. Keep your arms pressed down by your sides throughout the exercise.

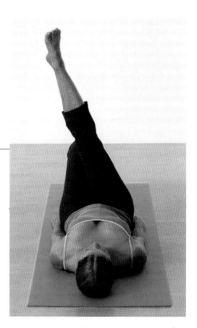

2 Inhale and, working the leg in Pilates stance (*see p21*), cross the right leg up and over your body, aiming for your left shoulder. Do not allow the right hip to lift up off the mat.

At a glance

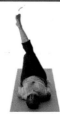
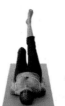
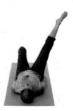
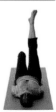

Inhale to circle down........................Exhale to circle up........Repeat

3 Sweep the leg down through the centre line of your body and out in line with your right shoulder.

4 Exhale and carry the leg back to the starting position. Circle 5 times in each direction, clockwise and anti-clockwise. Switch legs and repeat.

TRANSITION: *Bend the knee in and place both feet on the mat. Use the Preparation exercise (see pp26–27) to sit up at the edge of the mat for Rolling Like a Ball (see pp38–39).*

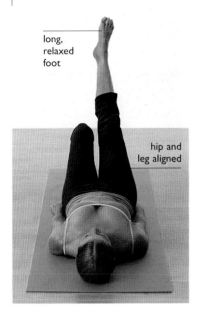

long, relaxed foot

hip and leg aligned

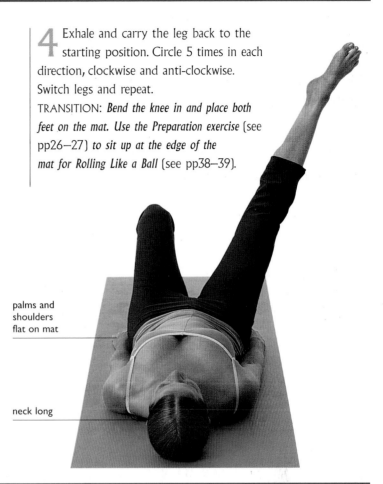

palms and shoulders flat on mat

neck long

HEAD-TO-TOE CHECKLIST

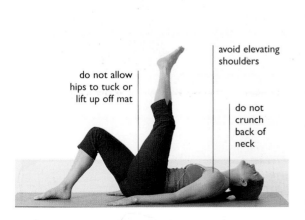

do not allow hips to tuck or lift up off mat

avoid elevating shoulders

do not crunch back of neck

- **Lengthen** the back of your neck by pressing your skull firmly into the mat. This will help you to pull your wings down.
- **Pin** your shoulders and arms down to the mat. Keep reaching the fingers long.
- **Control** your pelvis. Despite the circular movement of the leg, the hips should not shift or rock back and forth.
- **Do not** let the hips tuck (see p18) or lift up off the mat at any time.
- **Anchor** your bottom foot on the mat. Align the hip, knee, and foot and do not allow the knee to wave back and forth as you circle the leg.
- **Keep** the upper knee as straight as possible and work in Pilates stance.

ROLLING LIKE A BALL

This exercise begins to work the body dynamically. To execute properly, you will need to apply all the Pilates principles you have practised so far. Centre your body to control your "box" (*see p14*) and concentrate on precision and flow. The challenge is to move continuously without sacrificing your form or attention to detail.

REPETITIONS Repeat entire sequence 6–10 times.

CAUTION If you have a severe scoliosis, you may omit this exercise. Proceed with caution if you have a history of back injury.

VISUALIZATION Imagine imprinting an impression of your spine as you roll down, each vertebra making a small indentation on the mat underneath you.

1 Place your legs hip width apart and wrap your hands behind your thighs. Tip back and find your balance, curving the lower back.

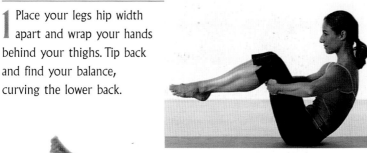

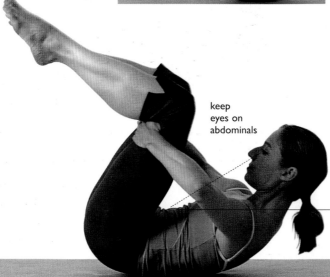

keep eyes on abdominals

2 Tilt the head down slightly and pull the abdominals into the spine. Keep your elbows lifted and inhale as you roll back onto the mat, just like a ball.

hollow out midsection

At a glance

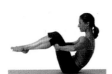 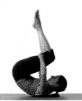 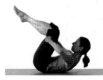 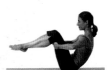

Inhale to roll back..Exhale to roll up........Repeat

3 Continue to roll back, lifting your hips until you reach the base of the shoulder blades. Without changing your shape, exhale and roll back up to your original Step 1 position. Repeat 6–10 times. TRANSITION: *Place your feet on the mat and your hands by your hips. Move back to the centre of the mat and lie back for the Single Leg Stretch* (see pp40–41).

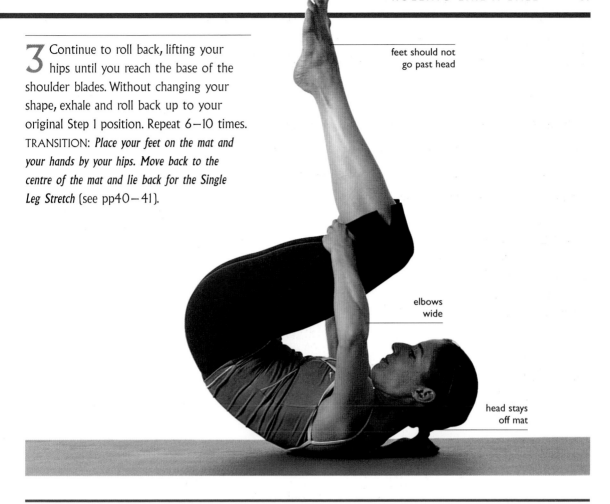

feet should not go past head

elbows wide

head stays off mat

HEAD-TO-TOE CHECKLIST

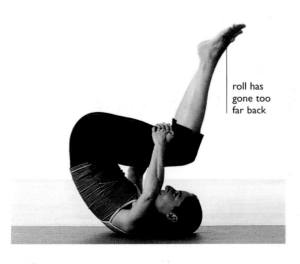

roll has gone too far back

• **Do not** roll onto your neck or let your head touch the mat.

• **Do not allow** the knees to pull in towards the chest when rolling back, or to pull away from the body when rolling up.

• **Never** let the feet open over the head.

• **Avoid** opening the knees away from you and straightening the arms, which will cause you to whip up from the bottom of the roll. Roll up only as far as you can; increase the work to the abdominals with each repetition.

• **If stiff** areas in your spine make it difficult to roll smoothly, try going slower. Roll quietly – your spine should not make any sound as it rolls on the mat.

SINGLE LEG STRETCH

Reciprocal movements add another dimension to your workout. This exercise requires you to move your legs while bracing your powerhouse. Work within your "frame" (*see p20*), aligning your shoulders and hips. Your legs move easily out and in, working toward the centre line of the body.

<table>
<tr><td>REPETITIONS 5–8 sets of alternating legs.</td></tr>
<tr><td>CAUTION If you have a knee injury, place your hands behind the knee rather than on top. If neck pain develops, rest your head.</td></tr>
<tr><td>VISUALIZATION Imagine a place in space and aim each foot for that spot – one foot replaces the other every time.</td></tr>
</table>

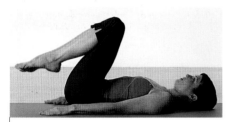

1 At the end of Rolling Like a Ball (*pp38–39*), move to the centre of the mat and lie back. Draw both knees in to your chest. Feel the back of your neck long and straight on the mat.

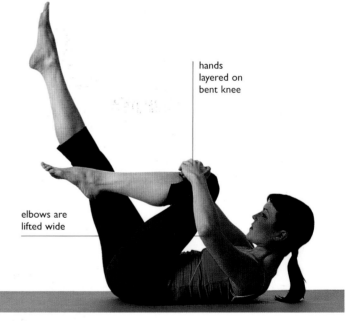

hands layered on bent knee

elbows are lifted wide

2 Lift up and pull one knee into the chest as you extend the other leg up towards the sky. The head and shoulders are off the mat and the elbows are wide. Hug the knee towards the shoulder, gently stretching.

At a glance

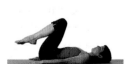 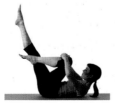 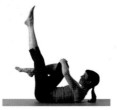 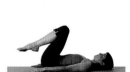

Inhale and exhale for alternate sets...Rest

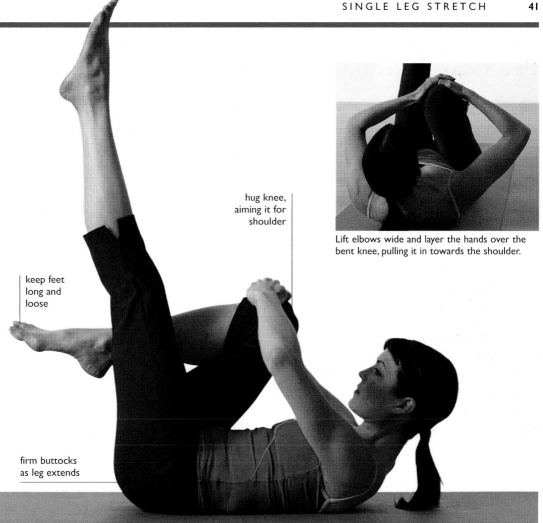

hug knee,
aiming it for
shoulder

Lift elbows wide and layer the hands over the
bent knee, pulling it in towards the shoulder.

keep feet
long and
loose

firm buttocks
as leg extends

3 Without disrupting your alignment, switch legs. Keep pulling the navel in towards the spine as you alternate legs, stretching one leg out as you hug the other knee in. Breathe in for one set and out for the next set. You may return to your Step 1 position to rest, or move on to the Transition.

TRANSITION: *Hug both knees in to the chest, bringing both hands onto the ankles for the Double Leg Stretch (see pp42–43). You may rest your head if necessary.*

HEAD-TO-TOE CHECKLIST

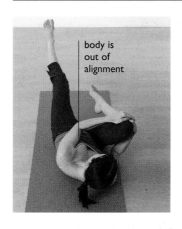

body is
out of
alignment

• **Avoid** rolling off one shoulder or hip – keep your box square.
• **Hug** the knee in to the body, maintaining perfect alignment – the hip, knee, and foot are all in one line.
• **Begin** with your upper leg towards the ceiling. As you improve, you may lower the leg to 45°.

DOUBLE LEG STRETCH

The Double Leg Stretch tests the powerhouse by moving the arms and legs simultaneously while the body remains still. There is an added element of breath to this exercise: keep the chin to the chest (*see p20*) and breathe fully and deeply, emptying the lungs completely with each exhalation.

REPETITIONS 5–8 times (Steps 2–3).

CAUTION If you experience neck pain while your head is up, you may rest it intermittently.

VISUALIZATION Imagine wringing the air out of your lungs the way you would wring out a wet towel.

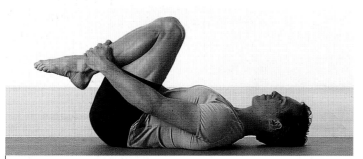

1 Begin with both knees drawn in to the chest and one hand on each ankle. If you chose to rest your head after the Single Leg Stretch (*see pp40–41*), re-establish your alignment and press the wings back and down.

2 Lift the head and shoulders off the mat and pull the chin towards the chest. Exhale as you hug the knees in, stretching the hips without allowing the buttocks or lower back to lift off the mat.

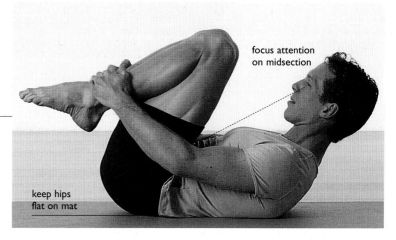

focus attention on midsection

keep hips flat on mat

At a glance

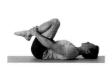 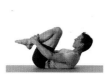 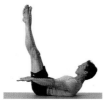 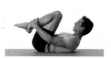 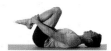

Breathe naturally...........Inhale to raise legs........Exhale to hug legs into chest

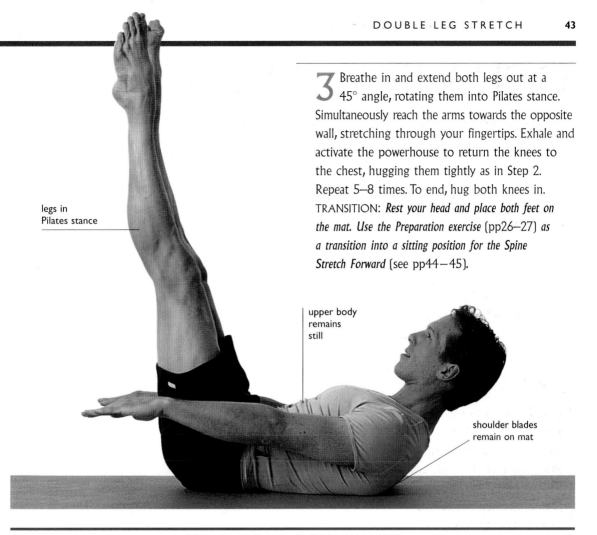

legs in
Pilates stance

3 Breathe in and extend both legs out at a 45° angle, rotating them into Pilates stance. Simultaneously reach the arms towards the opposite wall, stretching through your fingertips. Exhale and activate the powerhouse to return the knees to the chest, hugging them tightly as in Step 2. Repeat 5–8 times. To end, hug both knees in. TRANSITION: *Rest your head and place both feet on the mat. Use the Preparation exercise (pp26–27) as a transition into a sitting position for the Spine Stretch Forward (see pp44–45).*

upper body
remains
still

shoulder blades
remain on mat

HEAD-TO-TOE CHECKLIST

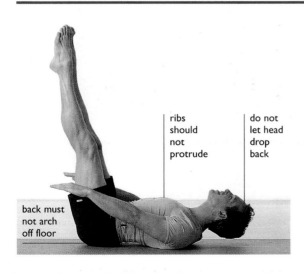

ribs
should
not
protrude

do not
let head
drop
back

back must
not arch
off floor

• **Keep** your chin towards your chest and eyes on your powerhouse. Do not let the head drop back.

• **Do not** let your legs extend too low – the lower back must remain solidly anchored on the floor throughout the entire sequence.

• **During Step 3**, anchor the upper body. Despite the continuous movement of your limbs, your torso should remain locked in position. Do not let your shoulders or upper back lift higher off the mat.

• Just as in the Single Leg Stretch, begin with your legs at a 90° angle. As you improve, you may lower the legs to 45°.

SPINE STRETCH FORWARD

This exercise, following on the heels of two challenging abdominal exercises, will open the muscles of the lower back and stretch the backs of the legs. Move fluidly, paying special attention to your posture and, as always, to the work of the powerhouse. This is the last exercise of the introductory mat series.

REPETITIONS Repeat entire sequence 3–5 times.

CAUTION If this stretch feels too intense in your lower back, simply reduce the range of motion. Begin with a small movement and gradually increase.

VISUALIZATION Envision sitting against a wall and peeling your spine up and down the wall, segment by segment.

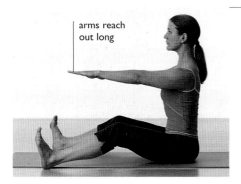

arms reach out long

1 Sit tall as though your back is against a wall. The legs are open and hip width apart, while the arms extend at shoulder height. Keep your knees soft and flex your feet.

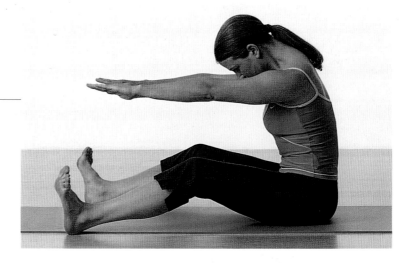

2 Exhale and lower your head as though you were diving through your arms. Round forwards with your upper back, leaving your lower back on the imaginary wall. Pull your navel in to the spine, stretching the lower back even further behind you.

At a glance

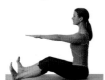
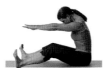
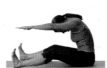

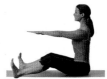

Inhale to begin.........Exhale to round over............................Inhale to sit tall

3 Increase the stretch by aiming the top of your head down towards the mat. Do not lower your arms. Continue to flex your feet, pulling your toes up. Inhale to reverse the motion, curling up to a tall, sitting position as in Step 1. Draw the abdominals in and up to establish your best posture.

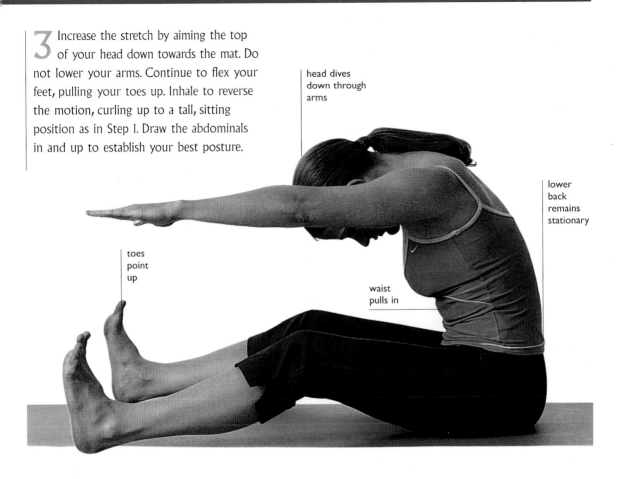

head dives down through arms

lower back remains stationary

toes point up

waist pulls in

HEAD-TO-TOE CHECKLIST

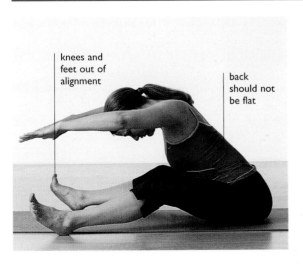

knees and feet out of alignment

back should not be flat

• **Use opposition** – the waist pulls behind you as the body reaches forwards.

• **Do not allow** your back to flatten. You may feel a deeper stretch in the backs of your legs by doing so, but this is not the area we are focusing on in this exercise.

• **During Step 2** firm your buttocks, lifting up higher off the mat.

• **Keep** your legs aligned. The toes point directly up to the ceiling.

• **Reach** the arms forwards to the opposite side of the room throughout.

• **Articulate** the spine when rolling back up to sit tall. Stack each vertebra, one above the other, until you are completely upright. Be careful not to lean back.

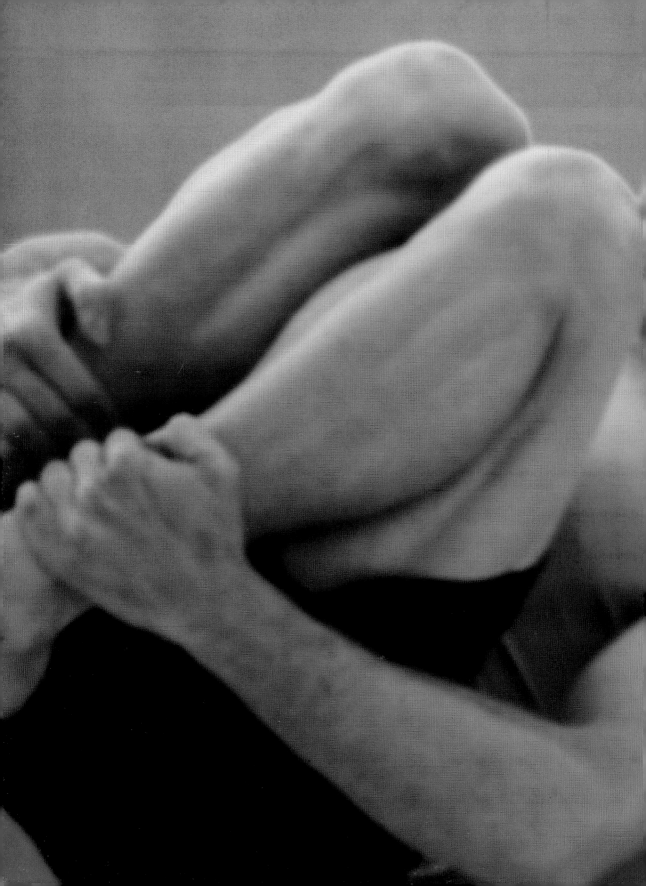

2

BEGINNER'S PROGRAMME

Slightly different in structure from the Introductory Programme, the beginner's syllabus focuses on the elements of *centring* and *control*. This chapter assumes a working knowledge of the basic principles and sets out to increase strength and speed within a framework of familiar exercises.

THE HUNDRED

The beginner Hundred builds on the work of the introductory version. In addition to increasing your endurance, you will also be required to sustain your legs at an angle, relying solely upon the strength of your powerhouse. Use your gluteal (buttock) muscles to create a support system for your lower back.

REPETITIONS 10 sets of full breath cycles (100 pumps).

CAUTION If you experience back pain while holding your legs up, refer back to the Introductory Hundred (pp32–33).

VISUALIZATION Imagine your arms beating out the tempo to a piece of music.

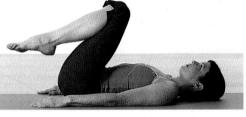

1 Lie flat on your back to begin, with both knees drawn in to the chest. Lengthen the back of the neck and slide your shoulders down and back.

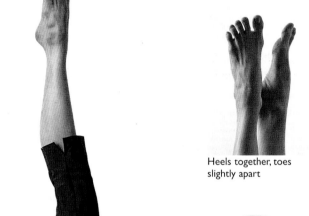

Heels together, toes slightly apart

chin to chest

2 Initiate from the abdominals to raise your head and shoulders, drawing the chin towards the chest. Stretch your arms long, past your hips, and straighten both legs up towards the ceiling. Rotate the legs into Pilates stance.

At a glance

  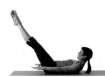

Inhale for 5 pumps...Exhale for 5 pumps

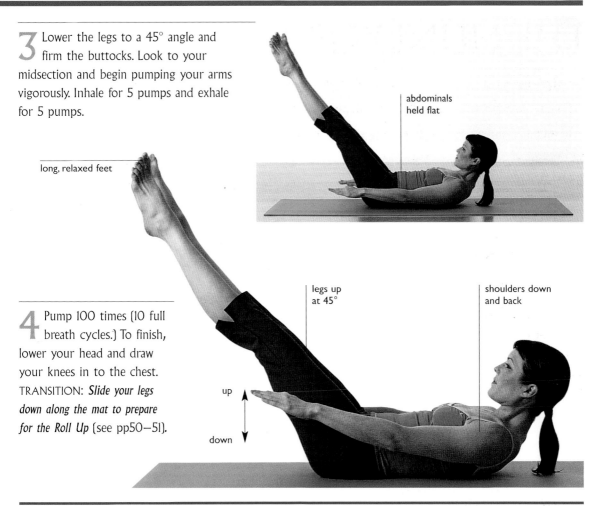

3 Lower the legs to a 45° angle and firm the buttocks. Look to your midsection and begin pumping your arms vigorously. Inhale for 5 pumps and exhale for 5 pumps.

abdominals held flat

long, relaxed feet

legs up at 45°

shoulders down and back

4 Pump 100 times (10 full breath cycles.) To finish, lower your head and draw your knees in to the chest. TRANSITION: *Slide your legs down along the mat to prepare for the Roll Up* (see pp50–51).

up

down

HEAD-TO-TOE CHECKLIST

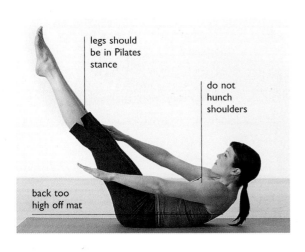

legs should be in Pilates stance

do not hunch shoulders

back too high off mat

• **Keep** shoulders down and back while pumping the arms.

• **Pump** the arms briskly, working about 25cm (6in) above the floor.

• **Do not** allow the motion of the arms to affect the rest of your body: the trunk and legs should remain still.

• **Breathe** in through your nose and out through your mouth.

• **You may not** be able to complete 10 sets initially. Begin with 5 sets and gradually increase the number of sets you can perform at one time.

ROLL UP

Although the Roll Up resembles a traditional "sit-up", it is not to be approached either speedily or carelessly. Here we demonstrate how one movement can simultaneously address strength, control, and flexibility. During the Roll Up you will work your spine in the same way as you did during the Preparation exercise (*see pp26–27*).

> **REPETITIONS** Repeat entire sequence 3–5 times.
>
> **CAUTION** Those with very weak abdominals may elect to continue performing the Roll Down (*pp34–35*) before attempting this exercise.
>
> **VISUALIZATION** Peel your spine up off the mat as if you were peeling a banana.

1 Lie flat on the mat and reach your arms overhead, just above your ears. Press the legs tightly together and flex your feet.

3 Breathe in and curl your body up off the mat as you aim your fingers towards your toes. Pull the powerhouse in and articulate each vertebra as the spine rolls slowly up.

2 Raise your arms up over your eyeline and bring your chin towards your chest. Look into your navel and do not allow it to bulge.

At a glance

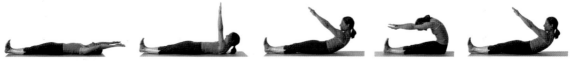

Inhale as you curl up off the mat.....Exhale to round over.....Inhale to curl back

4 Exhale and pull the waist in as you round over. Inhale as you pull your spine back down to the mat, sliding your pelvis underneath you. When your shoulders reach the mat, return the arms overhead.
TRANSITION: *Lower your arms to your sides for the Advanced Roll Over (pp116–119) or the Beginner Single Leg Circles (see pp52–53).*

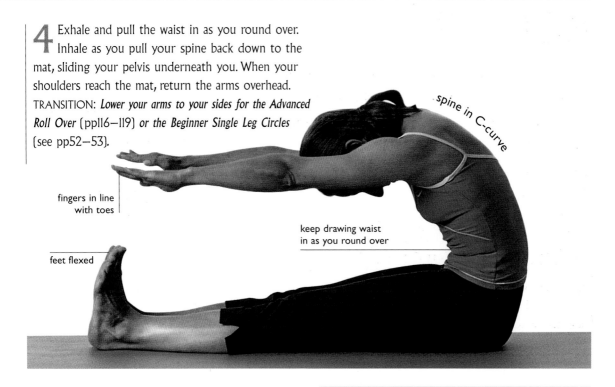

spine in C-curve

fingers in line with toes

keep drawing waist in as you round over

feet flexed

MODIFIED ROLL UP

To help you maintain your scoop and articulate through the spine, crawl your hands up alongside your legs – or anchor your feet under a piece of furniture.

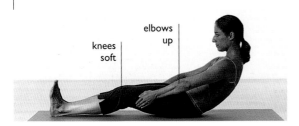

knees soft

elbows up

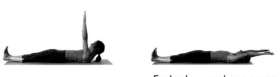

.............................Exhale and repeat

HEAD-TO-TOE CHECKLIST

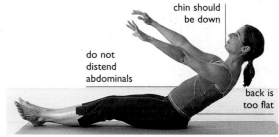

chin should be down

do not distend abdominals

back is too flat

• **During Step 1**, do not let the rib cage expand or the back arch off the mat as you reach overhead.
• **Keep** the chin down towards the chest.
• **Do not let** the abdominals protrude as you roll up.

• **Reach the** fingers just as far as the toes, not beyond them.
• **Lower** down to the mat, one vertebra at a time – first the lower back, then the middle back, and finally the upper back.

SINGLE LEG CIRCLES

Extending both legs for the beginner's Single Leg Circles further challenges the stability you have developed. Beyond strengthening the hip and stretching the back of the leg, this exercise also stretches and tones the outside of the thigh. Circle dynamically, stressing the "upswing" each time.

REPETITIONS 5 times in each direction, clockwise and anti-clockwise, with each leg.

CAUTION If you experience any clicking in your hip, rotate slightly and reduce the range of motion. If back pain occurs, refer back to the Introductory Single Leg Circles (pp36–37).

VISUALIZATION Imagine your leg slicing through the air in a perfect circle.

1 Following the Roll Up (*see pp50–51*), draw the right leg in and straighten it up to the ceiling. Square your box and anchor your powerhouse.

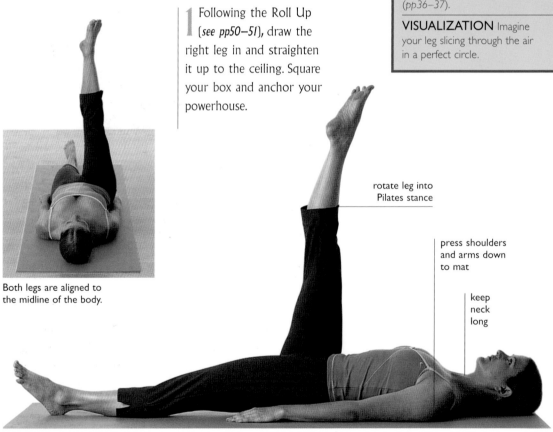

Both legs are aligned to the midline of the body.

rotate leg into Pilates stance

press shoulders and arms down to mat

keep neck long

At a glance

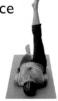 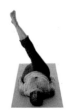 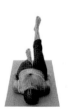 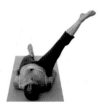 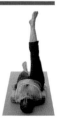

Inhale for one set.............Exhale for next set.......................Repeat

2 Breathe in and begin drawing the arc of a circle. Aim your heel for your opposite shoulder so that the motion of the leg is "up and across". Steady your hips on the mat as the leg moves.

3 In a continuous, sweeping motion, take the leg down towards the midline. Do not allow the back to arch up off the mat. Continue moving the leg onto the second half of the circle.

4 Glide the leg out and back to the starting position, emphasizing the upswing as you exhale. Repeat the circling 5 times then reverse direction for 5 more. Switch legs and repeat the entire sequence.
TRANSITION: *Hug knee to the chest then slide it down next to other leg. Roll up to sitting and use your hands to lift your bottom to the front of the mat for Rolling Like a Ball (see pp54–55).*

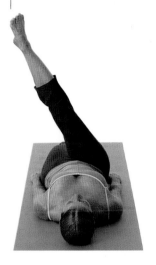

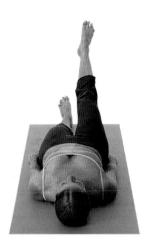

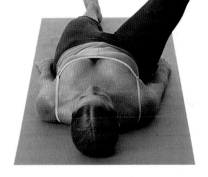

HEAD-TO-TOE CHECKLIST

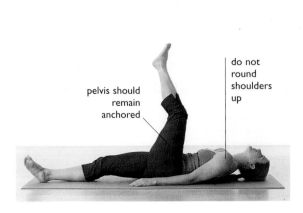

pelvis should remain anchored

do not round shoulders up

- **Avoid** lifting the chin and crunching the back of the neck.
- **Press** the back of the neck, the shoulders, and the arms firmly into the mat during the exercise.
- **Draw** the navel in and up, hollowing out your midsection.
- **The circling leg** is rotated into Pilates stance.

- **The bottom leg** reaches out and away from body.
- **Stretch** the knees as much as possible.
- **Circle** the leg energetically, but do not use momentum.
- **Ensure** that your body remains solidly positioned on the mat. The motion of the leg should not cause you to roll off to one side.

ROLLING LIKE A BALL

This exercise is the one you are most likely to "cheat" your way through. Performed at the proper tempo, your muscles will work to their threshold. If you roll too quickly, the benefits of the exercise are lost. Pay close attention to your form, adjusting your rhythm and position in order to challenge yourself.

REPETITIONS Repeat entire sequence 6–10 times.

CAUTION If you have a severe scoliosis, you may omit this exercise. Use discretion if you have a history of back injury.

VISUALIZATION Imagine you have been stuffed inside a bubble. If you lose your "ball" shape, you'll pop the bubble.

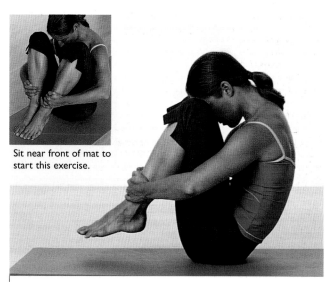

Sit near front of mat to start this exercise.

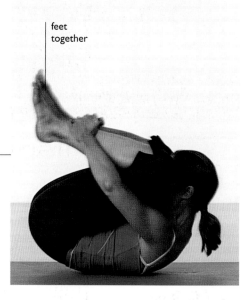

feet together

1 Balance on your sit-bones and clutch one ankle in each hand. Pull your feet close to your buttocks and place your head squarely between your knees.

2 Inhale and roll back on the mat, keeping your shape uniform. The feet should stay close to the buttocks, while the head remains between the knees.

At a glance

Inhale to roll back......................................Exhale to roll up...............Repeat

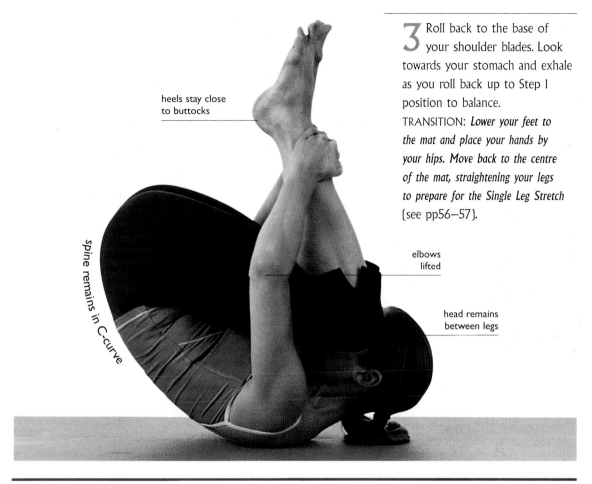

heels stay close
to buttocks

spine remains in C-curve

elbows
lifted

head remains
between legs

3 Roll back to the base of your shoulder blades. Look towards your stomach and exhale as you roll back up to Step 1 position to balance.

TRANSITION: *Lower your feet to the mat and place your hands by your hips. Move back to the centre of the mat, straightening your legs to prepare for the Single Leg Stretch (see pp56–57).*

HEAD-TO-TOE CHECKLIST

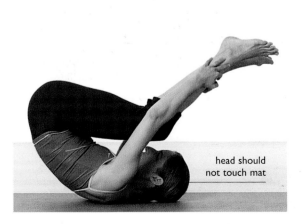

head should
not touch mat

- **Start** this exercise sitting at the front of the mat to allow yourself room to roll back and forth.
- **Never roll** onto your neck or allow your head to touch the mat.
- **Keep** the shoulders relaxed throughout.
- **The head** must remain between the knees, especially when rolling up.
- **Avoid** using momentum.

Do not roll up too fast and then sit tall, flattening the spine. Keep your C-curve active and your navel drawn in to your spine – particularly at the balance point.

- **You may** not be able to roll all the way back up initially. In this case, do not sacrifice your form. Simply roll up as high as you can and continue to practise.

SINGLE LEG STRETCH

With the torso locked in place and the limbs moving freely, this exercise will strengthen the abdominals and the buttocks as well as improve coordination. It is the first of five exercises commonly termed the Stomach Series: these may be done independently of the rest of the mat programme for a quick workout.

REPETITIONS 5–10 sets of alternating legs.

CAUTION Should you experience knee pain, simply hold under the knee and continue.

VISUALIZATION Imagine looking down on yourself from the ceiling. Keep your alignment perfect, your box square, and your legs in line.

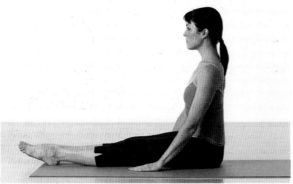

After Rolling Like a Ball (see pp54–55), use your hands to lift your buttocks back to the centre of the mat.

1 Lower your chin to your chest and roll yourself down to the mat, articulating each vertebra one by one. Lie flat and position yourself squarely in the centre of the mat.

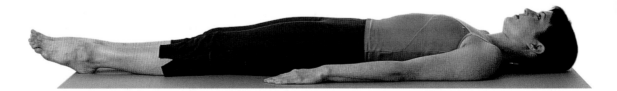

At a glance

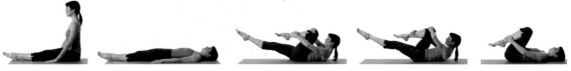

Inhale for one set.........................Exhale for next set............................Rest

2 Lift your head and shoulders off the mat. Hug the left knee in and extend the right leg out to 45°. The left hand holds the left ankle and the right hand holds the left knee.

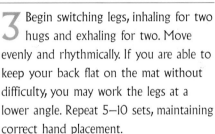

The outside hand holds the ankle while the inside hand holds the knee.

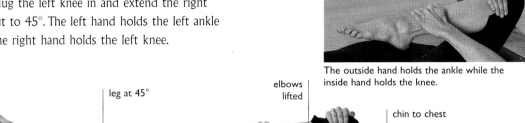

leg at 45°

elbows lifted

chin to chest

tight buttocks

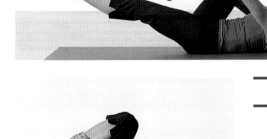

3 Begin switching legs, inhaling for two hugs and exhaling for two. Move evenly and rhythmically. If you are able to keep your back flat on the mat without difficulty, you may work the legs at a lower angle. Repeat 5–10 sets, maintaining correct hand placement.

HEAD-TO-TOE CHECKLIST

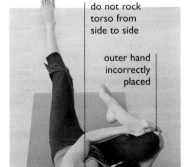

do not rock torso from side to side

outer hand incorrectly placed

• **Keep** your box square and focus on the midline. Do not rock your body from side to side when switching legs.

• **Pay attention** to the hand placement, which keeps your legs well aligned.

• **Squeeze** your buttocks each time the leg stretches out.

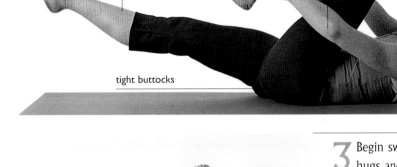

4 To finish, hug both knees in towards the chest.

TRANSITION: *You may rest your head only if necessary. Otherwise leave it up and move directly into the Double Leg Stretch* (see pp58–59).

DOUBLE LEG STRETCH

As the second exercise in the Stomach Series, the beginner's Double Leg Stretch continues to challenge your coordination and your centre. The powerhouse will provide a base for your limbs, which simultaneously lengthen away from the centre of the body. Focus on the circular action of the arms and the specific breathing pattern.

REPETITIONS 5–10 times (Steps 2–4).

CAUTION Proceed with caution if you have back or disc injuries. Abbreviate the arm movement if you have a delicate shoulder.

VISUALIZATION Imagine the centre of your body thinning out like a rubber band as you stretch your body long and thin.

1 Following the Single Leg Stretch (*see pp56–57*), hug both knees in to the chest, bringing one hand to each ankle. If your head is down, check your alignment before moving on.

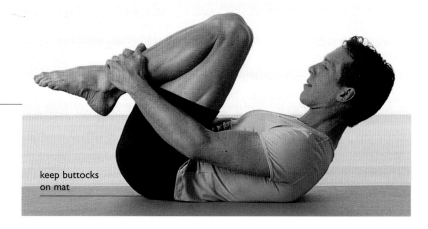

keep buttocks on mat

2 Lift your head and shoulders off the mat, using your powerhouse to sustain the position. Feel your lower back lengthening underneath you.

At a glance

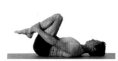 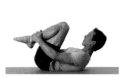 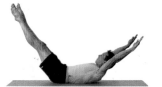 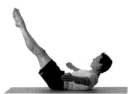

Inhale as arms and legs reach out......................Exhale as arms sweep around

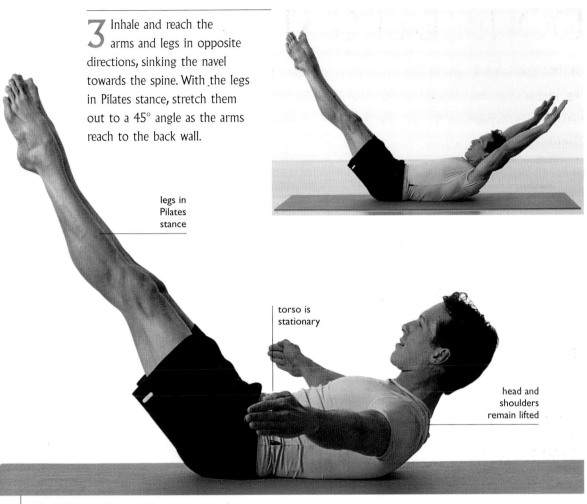

3 Inhale and reach the arms and legs in opposite directions, sinking the navel towards the spine. With the legs in Pilates stance, stretch them out to a 45° angle as the arms reach to the back wall.

legs in Pilates stance

torso is stationary

head and shoulders remain lifted

4 Exhale and sweep the arms around, then hug the knees tightly and repeat. Return to Step 1 position to end.

TRANSITION: *For the Intermediate and Advanced programmes, move into the Single Straight Leg Stretch (see pp74–75); or sit tall for the Beginner Spine Stretch Forward (see pp60–61).*

HEAD-TO-TOE CHECKLIST

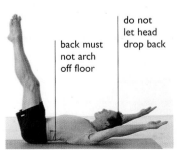

back must not arch off floor

do not let head drop back

• **Do not lower** the head and shoulders as you reach the arms back. Your torso must remain locked in position as your limbs move.
• **Ensure** that the lower back remains anchored to the floor throughout.
• **You may** begin with the legs at a 90° angle and gradually advance to 45°.

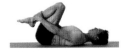

. . . . Rest

SPINE STRETCH FORWARD

The beginner's Spine Stretch Forward develops the work you did in the introductory version (*see pp44–45*). As this is the last exercise of the beginner series, focus on integrating all the principles of the earlier exercises. Here, postural awareness, deep breathing, and the articulation of the spine are combined with a generous stretch.

REPETITIONS Repeat entire sequence 3–5 times.

CAUTION If you find the stretch behind the knees too intense, soften the legs and keep the thigh muscles relaxed.

VISUALIZATION Imagine moulding your body into the shape of a huge horseshoe.

arms parallel to legs

1 Sit upright with the navel pulled in and up. Your legs should be hip width apart with the feet flexed, while the arms are lifted parallel to the legs.

2 Firm the buttocks and begin to round up and over. Keep your lower back pressing behind you and hollow out the abdominals.

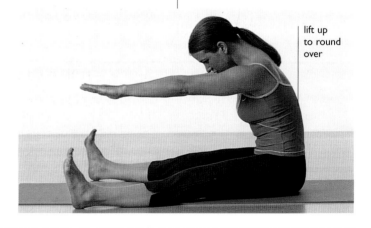

lift up to round over

At a glance

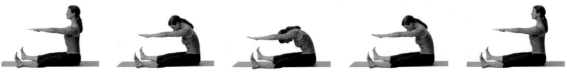

Inhale to sit tall...........Exhale to round over.....................................Inhale

3 Deepen the curve of the spine while increasing the scoop in the navel. Reverse the motion, rolling back up to Step 1 position, stacking one vertebra at a time.

TRANSITION: *Bend your knees and draw both ankles in towards your centre for the Intermediate Open Leg Rocker (see pp82–83) or the Intermediate Open Leg Rocker Preparation (see pp80–81), or you may finish here.*

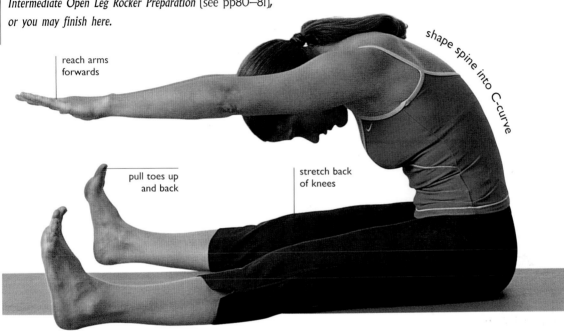

reach arms forwards

shape spine into C-curve

pull toes up and back

stretch back of knees

HEAD-TO-TOE CHECKLIST

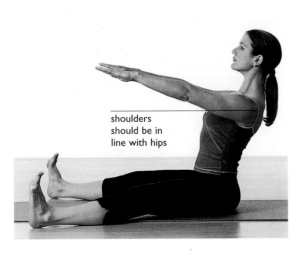

shoulders should be in line with hips

- **Resist** slumping down or hinging forwards at the hips, which can cause the stomach muscles to relax. The abdominals must pull in towards the spine.
- **Allow** your head to hang loosely down at the bottom of the stretch.
- **Continue** to push out through your heels, stretching the backs of your legs throughout.

- **Roll back up** to perfect posture, being careful to align your shoulders over your hips – do not lean forwards or back.
- **As you sit tall** press your wings down and lengthen your neck.
- **During Step 2**, begin by tightening the gluteals and lifting up higher in the waist to round forwards.

THE WALL

The Wall Series helps to transfer our bodies from the mat to the upright posture of daily life. It may be performed separately from your workout — use it to refresh, realign, and rejuvenate yourself.

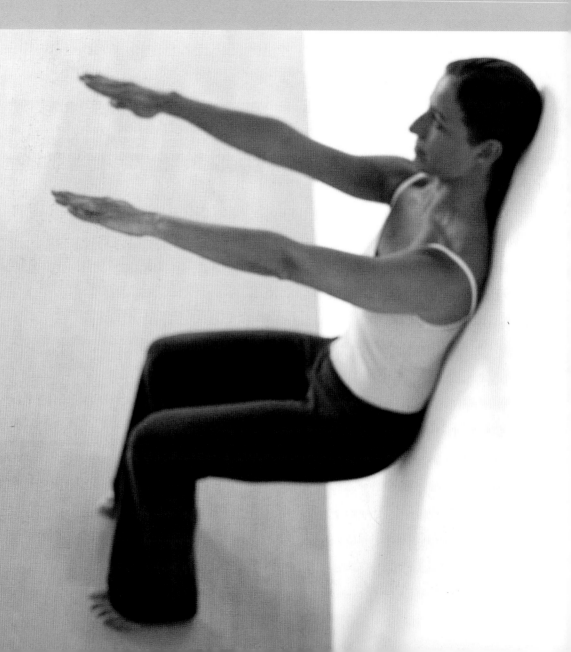

THE WALL: STANDING

Posture is the basis of all of our movements and, in many ways, our wellbeing is reflected in how we stand and walk. The Wall is a tool to make us aware of our postural habits and to help us improve them. We begin with a basic standing exercise to establish correct alignment.

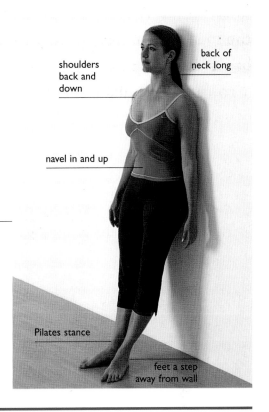

shoulders back and down

back of neck long

navel in and up

Stand against a wall, with your feet about one step away. The legs work in Pilates stance. Align your spine firmly against the wall from your tailbone to the back of your head. Draw the navel in and up and breathe naturally. Remain standing for several moments, perfecting your posture. TRANSITION: *Move directly on to the Wall: Arm Circles* (see p64).

Pilates stance

feet a step away from wall

HEAD-TO-TOE CHECKLIST

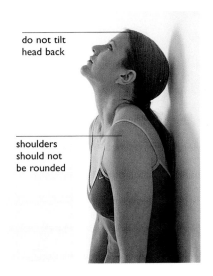

do not tilt head back

shoulders should not be rounded

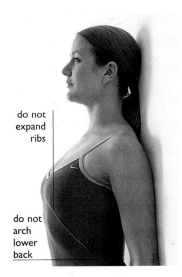

do not expand ribs

do not arch lower back

• **Do not** lift the chin in an effort to get the back of your head against the wall. Think of slightly tucking the chin in to lengthen the back of the neck, even if the head does not press against the wall.

• **Keep the chest** lifted and the shoulders back.

• **Work** to keep the lower back flush against the wall. You may need to soften your knees slightly.

THE WALL: ARM CIRCLES

The work of the Wall is to reeducate your spine and establish improved postural alignment. Having practised this in the Wall: Standing exercise (*see p63*), we move on to the Arm Circles to reinforce the concept of controlled mobility. Remember, all movement flows outwards from a strong centre.

1 From the Wall: Standing position, hold yourself solidly against the wall, from head to tail. Take a few deep breaths. Open the chest and press the shoulders back while the arms hang loosely by your sides.

2 Keep the back of your neck long and raise both arms to shoulder height in front of the body. Draw the abdominals in even deeper, pressing into the small of your back without pulling your upper back or shoulders away from the wall.

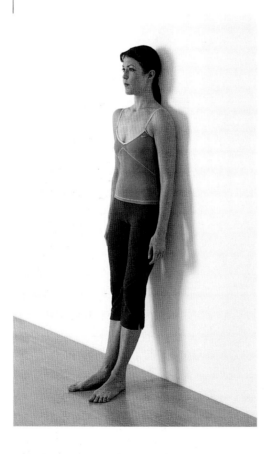

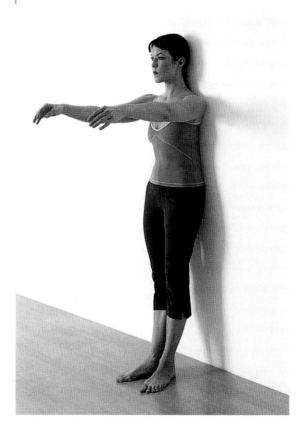

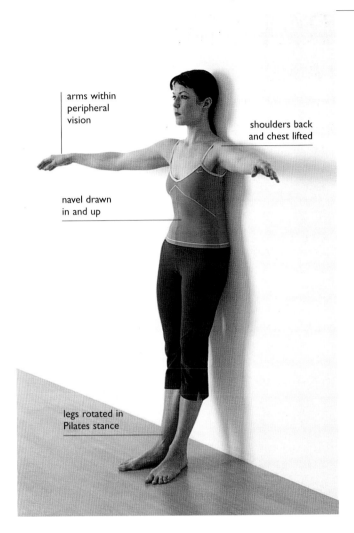

arms within
peripheral
vision

shoulders back
and chest lifted

navel drawn
in and up

legs rotated in
Pilates stance

3 Open the arms within your peripheral vision. The navel continues to draw in and up. Your neck stretches long behind you.

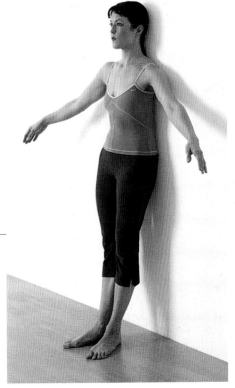

4 Lower the arms to complete the circle just in front of your thighs. Repeat 3 circles each way, breathing naturally. If you cannot maintain the back of your head or shoulders against the wall without lifting the chin, simply leave it off the wall, but check that it is in line with the rest of your spine. TRANSITION: *To end, move directly into the Wall: Roll Down (see pp66–67).*

THE WALL: ROLL DOWN

The Wall Series continues with a spinal articulation exercise. Without gravity to assist you, as in the matwork, spinal mobility is more challenging. Work your spine as though you were a stegosaurus dinosaur with spokes running up and down your back: take one spoke off the wall at a time and replace them as you roll up.

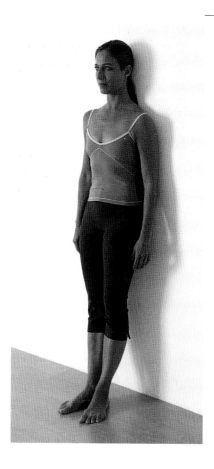

1 Establish your position with your feet one step away from the wall. Press the entire length of the spine, from the back of your head to your buttocks, firmly into the wall. If you have difficulty getting the back of your head against the wall without tilting it back, leave it off the wall but aligned with the rest of your spine.

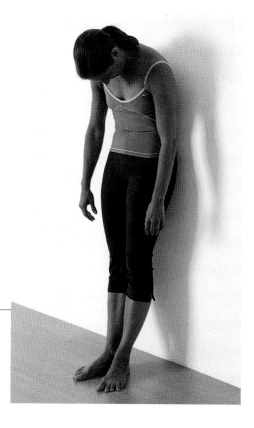

2 Begin peeling off the wall. Drop the head first, then the shoulders. Relax the arms loosely at your sides. Continue to pull the waist up and feel your lower back pushing the wall away.

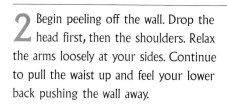

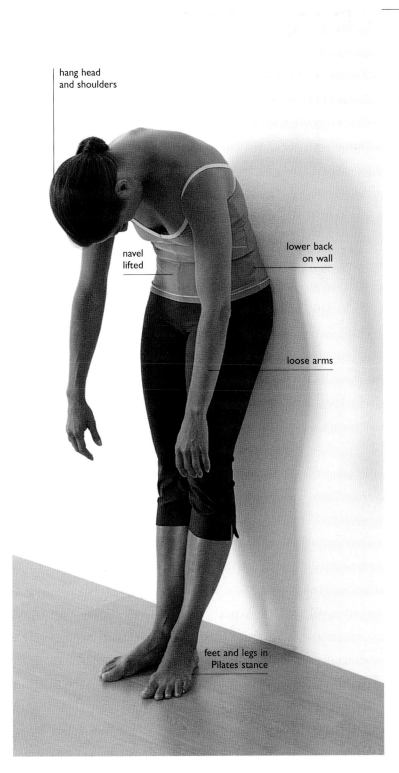

hang head
and shoulders

navel
lifted

lower back
on wall

loose arms

feet and legs in
Pilates stance

3 Increase the rolling down, peeling the ribs off the wall but pulling the navel up higher. The head and arms hang freely. Circle the arms 4 times in each direction, clockwise and anti-clockwise. Reverse the roll down, coming up vertebra by vertebra until you have returned to the starting position. Repeat the exercise 1–2 times.

TRANSITION: *Move directly on to the Wall: The Chair* (see pp68–69).

CAUTION If this exercise causes strain to your neck or shoulders, work only within a pain-free range. You may also initiate the exercise with your head away from the wall.

THE WALL: THE CHAIR

The last exercise in the series, the Chair is akin to the wall slides traditionally performed to strengthen the quadriceps or upper thigh muscles. When done Pilates-style, we add elements of posture and spinal alignment as well as abdominal power. This is the final exercise in the **Wall Series**.

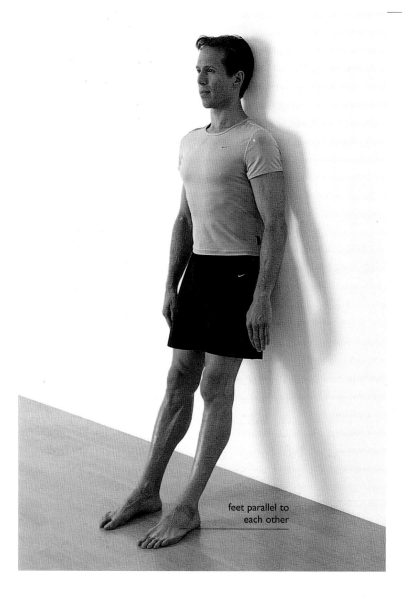

feet parallel to each other

1 Begin standing against the wall, your feet one large step away. Align your legs in parallel with the hips, knees, and feet all pointing straight ahead. The neck lengthens as you press the base of the skull into the wall. Open the chest and press the shoulders back towards the wall without allowing the ribs to protrude. The abdominals draw in and up.

CAUTION If you experience any knee pain during this exercise, eliminate it from your programme.

2 Bend the knees and simultaneously raise your arms. Lower down until the hips and knees are at 90° angles. The arms reach to the opposite side of the room, parallel with the legs. Breathe naturally and sustain this position for 3–5 counts. Pull your abdominals in and up and slide back up, keeping your hips in contact with the wall. As you rise up, lower your arms to their starting position. Repeat the exercise 2–3 times.

TRANSITION: *Bring one foot all the way back, pressing your heel into the wall. Without leaning forwards, press your palms into the wall and push off to a tall, standing posture. You have now completed the Wall Series.*

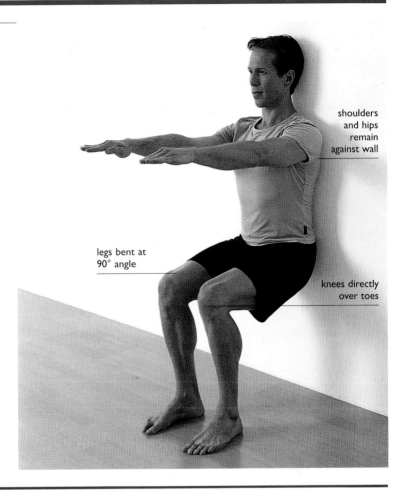

shoulders and hips remain against wall

legs bent at 90° angle

knees directly over toes

HEAD-TO-TOE CHECKLIST

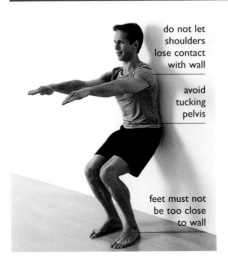

do not let shoulders lose contact with wall

avoid tucking pelvis

feet must not be too close to wall

• **The shoulders** and the head should keep contact with the wall throughout the exercise.

• **Avoid** tucking your pelvis underneath you. The entire length of your spine, including the tailbone, should remain against the wall as you slide up and down.

• **Place your feet** a good distance from the wall. As you reach the deepest point in the bend, your knees should be directly over your toes, not beyond them.

• **At the lowest** point, your body should look as though it is seated in a chair.

• **Slide up** the wall, initiating from your powerhouse. Move smoothly and avoid any jerking movements.

• **If sustaining** Step 2 position for three counts is too difficult, begin with one count and increase as you gain strength.

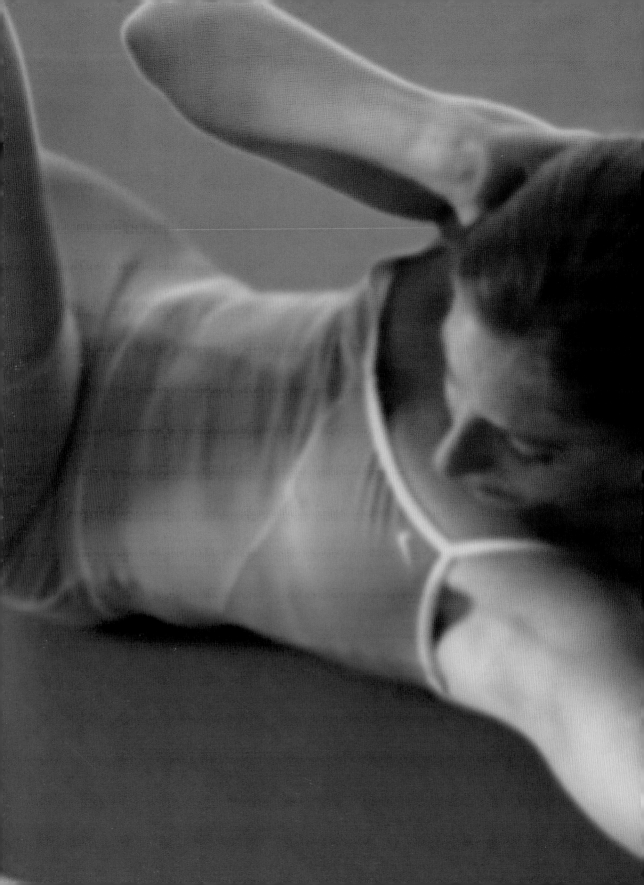

3

INTERMEDIATE PROGRAMME

This chapter introduces several new exercises. Positions change frequently and exercises now become more complex. Continue to fine-tune the movements you know and to practise what you find challenging. *Precision* is the focal point.

EXERCISE SEQUENCE

Building on the exercises in the preceding chapter, the Intermediate Programme adds several new exercises to your workout. This exercise sequence chart provides a visual cue card: when performed in the order shown, the entire programme will flow smoothly and easily. As you progress, you should need to refer only to the chart to complete your workout.

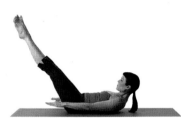

1 The Hundred
(pp48–49)

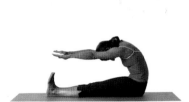

2 Roll Up
(pp50–51)

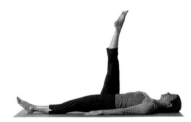

3 Single Leg Circles
(pp52–53)

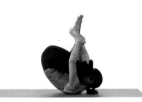

4 Rolling Like a Ball
(pp54–55)

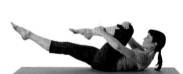

5 Single Leg Stretch
(pp56–57)

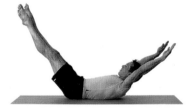

6 Double Leg Stretch
(pp58–59)

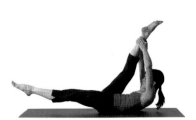

7 Single Straight Leg Stretch
(pp74–75)

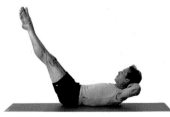

8 Double Straight Leg Stretch
(pp76–77)

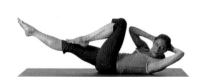

9 Criss-Cross
(pp78–79)

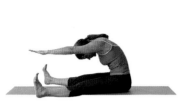

10 Spine Stretch Forward
(pp60–61)

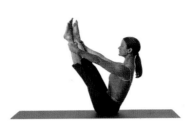

11 Open Leg Rocker
(pp80–83)

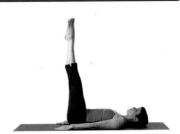

12 Corkscrew
(pp84–85)

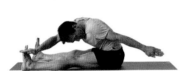

13 Saw
(pp86–87)

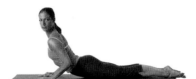

14 Neck Roll
(pp88–89)

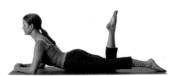

15 Single Leg Kick
(pp90–91)

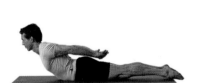

16 Double Leg Kick
(pp92–93)

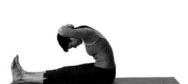

17 Neck Pull
(pp94–97)

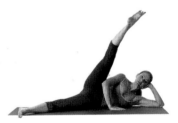

18 Side Kicks Series
(pp98–105)

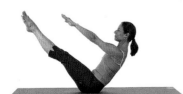

19 Teaser Series
(pp106–109)

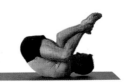

20 Seal
(pp110–111)

SINGLE STRAIGHT LEG STRETCH

The third exercise in the Stomach Series is also known as the "Scissors". It requires you to move quickly and with control. Once you feel comfortable with the mechanics, this exercise should be done as briskly as possible and with large sweeping movements of the legs. Work on holding your torso stable and your legs straight.

REPETITIONS 5–10 sets of alternating legs.

CAUTION If you develop neck pain while holding your head up during this exercise, you may rest it intermittently.

VISUALIZATION As you begin switching legs, imagine pulsing your legs in rhythm with your heartbeat.

1 The end of the Double Leg Stretch (*see pp58–59*) is the beginning of this exercise. Lying flat on the mat, hug your knees in to your chest and keep your head and shoulders curled up off the floor. The elbows are wide.

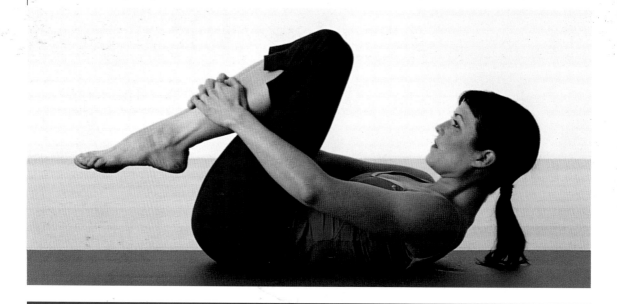

At a glance

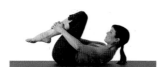
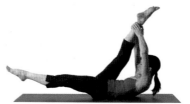
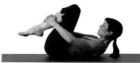

Breathe naturally.......... Inhale/Exhale for alternate sets........................Rest

2 Taking hold of the ankle, extend one leg up and stretch the opposite leg out. Use the hands to lightly pulse the top leg twice. Sink the navel deeper as the leg nears the body. Switch legs without jarring the upper body and repeat 5–10 sets. Return to Step 1 position to finish or move onto the Transition.

TRANSITION: *Bring the legs up to 90° and place both hands behind your head to prepare for the Double Straight Leg Stretch* (see pp76–77).

elbows are held wide

keep knees as straight as possible

legs reach towards midline of body

HEAD-TO-TOE CHECKLIST

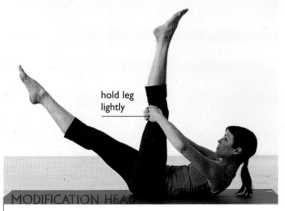

hold leg lightly

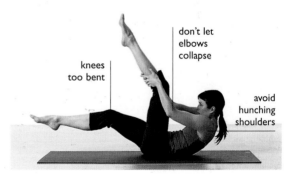

knees too bent

don't let elbows collapse

avoid hunching shoulders

MODIFIED STRETCH

If you cannot hold your ankle, simply adjust your hand placement, moving your hands up your leg towards your thigh. If you cannot hold any lower down than the knee, hold very lightly. Reduce the range of motion and scissor the legs within a pain-free range.

• **Avoid** the tendency to rock or bounce your body as the legs switch.

• **Do not ignore** the bottom leg. Reach it long and use Pilates stance to engage the buttocks.

• **Do not lift** your body up to your leg. Instead, bring the leg to you.

• **Keep** the neck and shoulders relaxed.

• **Deepen** the scoop as each leg scissors.

DOUBLE STRAIGHT LEG STRETCH

The Double Straight Leg Stretch reinforces the "controlled mobility" principle (*see p16*). The powerhouse holds the upper body stable as the legs smoothly reach down and up. Begin with small movements and engage the buttocks and inner thighs to support and protect your back.

REPETITIONS 5–10 times (Steps 2–3).

CAUTION Do not attempt this exercise if you have a weak back or a history of back injury. If you have a delicate neck, you may leave your head down.

VISUALIZATION Imagine your legs working like a windshield wiper, pressing down slowly and pulling up quickly.

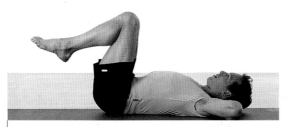

1 Lie on your back with both hands behind your head. Layer one hand over the other, ensuring that the fingers are not laced (*see detail*). Keep your elbows wide and anchor your torso to the mat throughout the sequence.

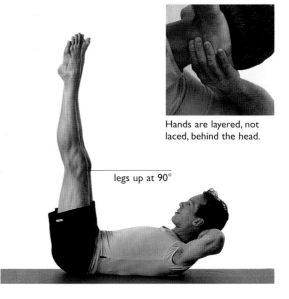

Hands are layered, not laced, behind the head.

legs up at 90°

2 Use your powerhouse to peel your head and shoulders up off the mat, focusing your eyes on your midsection. Extend both legs straight up into Pilates stance. Sink your navel towards the spine.

At a glance

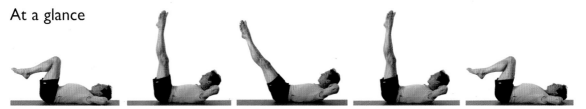

Breathe naturally..........Inhale to lower legs..........Exhale to lift legs........Rest

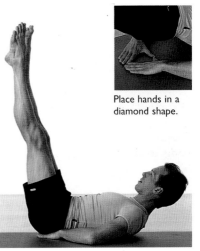

Place hands in a diamond shape.

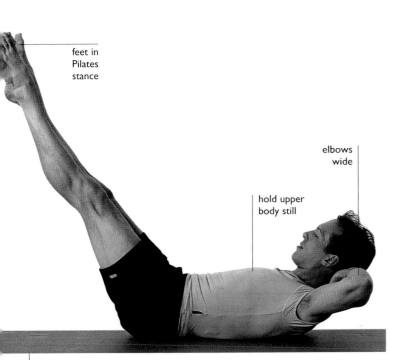

feet in Pilates stance

elbows wide

hold upper body still

3 Inhale and slowly reach your legs away from you for 3 counts. Exhale and return the legs to the ceiling in one swift motion. Repeat 5–10 times. Return to Step 1 position only if you need to rest. TRANSITION: *Keep your upper body elevated and bend both knees in to the chest to prepare for the Criss–Cross* (pp78–79).

ALTERNATIVE HAND POSITION

If you have a delicate back or experience any back pain while performing this exercise, place' your hands as shown to brace the lower back. In this position, press the elbows down to the mat and continue with the exercise.

HEAD-TO-TOE CHECKLIST

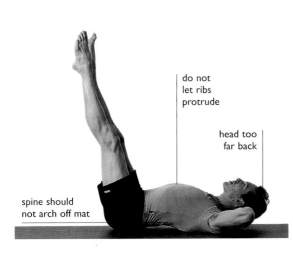

do not let ribs protrude

head too far back

spine should not arch off mat

• **If your back** arches off the mat as you lower your legs, you are taking them too low. Lower your legs only to your point of control. As your level of control improves, you may lower the legs further.

• **Do not allow** your legs to go past perpendicular or 90° when raising them. In addition, the buttocks must never rise off the mat as you return your legs to the ceiling.

• **Check** that you are initiating from the abdominals to move the legs and not relying on speed or momentum.

• **As the legs** move up and down, do not distend the abdominals. Instead, hold the ribs in firmly to keep your girdle area flat.

CRISS-CROSS

The final exercise of the Stomach Series targets the obliques or the diagonal muscles of the waist and trunk. Somewhat reminiscent of the old-style "bicycle" done in the gym, the Criss-Cross is executed slowly and smoothly with exacting detail. If you don't have time for a full mat workout, you can always do just the Stomach Series.

REPETITIONS 3–5 sets of alternating legs.

CAUTION Avoid twisting exercises such as this if you have suffered a recent back injury.

VISUALIZATION Imagine a magnetic force lifting your upper body directly up towards your bent knee.

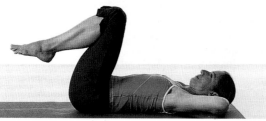

1 From the Double Straight Leg Stretch (*pp76–77*), keep the hands behind the head and draw the knees in to the body. If you choose to rest the head, do so briefly then move on to Step 2.

2 Inhale and rise up, twisting to one side as you extend one leg out. Aim the front elbow for the opposite knee and open the back elbow behind you. Hold for 3 counts.

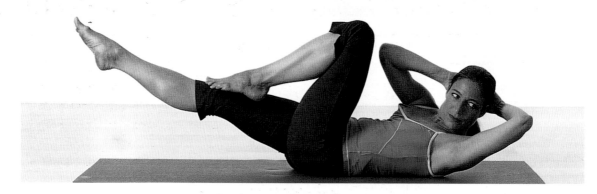

At a glance

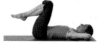 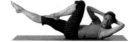 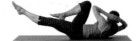 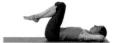

Inhale to criss..Exhale to cross.......Rest and repeat

3 Exhale and switch sides, holding for another 3 counts. Be certain not to lower your upper back as you pass through the centre. Repeat 3–5 sets and return to Step 1 position to rest

TRANSITION: *Release your hands and place both feet on the mat. Use the Preparation exercise (see pp26–27) to rise up for the Beginner Spine Stretch Forward (see pp60–61).*

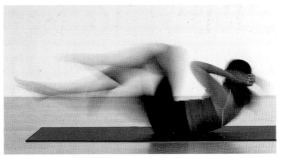

Keep your upper back and shoulders elevated off the mat as you twist from side to side.

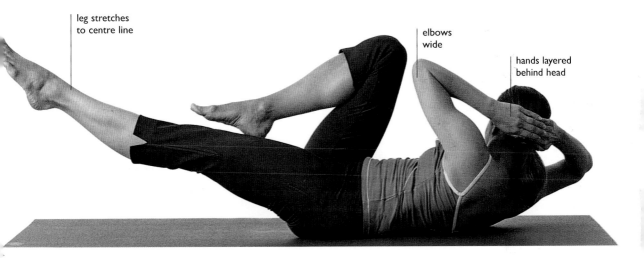

leg stretches to centre line

elbows wide

hands layered behind head

HEAD-TO-TOE CHECKLIST

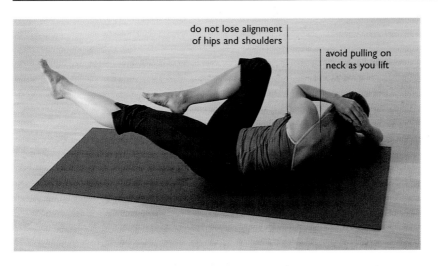

do not lose alignment of hips and shoulders

avoid pulling on neck as you lift

• **Never** pull on your neck. Lift from the powerhouse.

• **The back elbow** never touches the mat. Look towards it as you open it behind you.

• **Maintain** your "box". Hips and shoulders are square.

• **As you twist** avoid rolling from side to side.

• **Focus** on lengthening one side of the waist as you contract the other.

OPEN LEG ROCKER PREPARATION

To ready ourselves for the Open Leg Rocker (*see pp82–83*), we begin with a preparatory exercise. The objective here is to move the arms and legs in a continuous motion as well as in several directions, without disrupting your balance. The key to success is keeping your pelvis tipped back just far enough.

REPETITIONS Repeat first two steps 2–3 times then repeat entire sequence 2–3 times.

CAUTION A sensitive tailbone may be further irritated by this exercise. Proceed with caution.

VISUALIZATION Imagine strings attached to your ankles controlling the movements of your legs, just like a marionette.

Bring your hands inside the legs and grasp the ankles.

1 Scoop the belly in and balance on your tailbone, allowing your feet to hover just above the mat. Keep pressing the wings down and pulling the belly button in towards the backbone.

At a glance

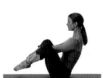

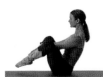

Inhale . . . . Exhale . . . . Inhale . . . . Exhale . . . . Inhale

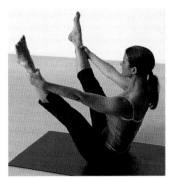

Following Step 1, the legs extend directly up to an open position.

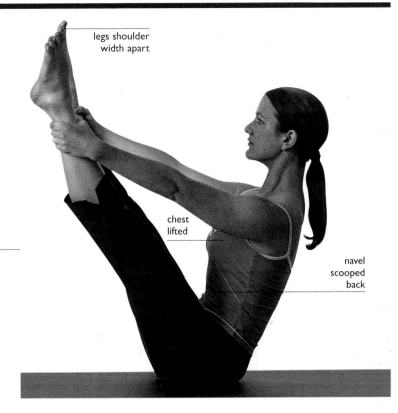

legs shoulder width apart

chest lifted

navel scooped back

2 Inhale and extend both legs up as straight as possible, shoulder width apart. Do not let the upper body collapse. Exhale to lower the legs to the Step 1 position. Repeat 2–3 times. Extend the legs one last time and hold them up.

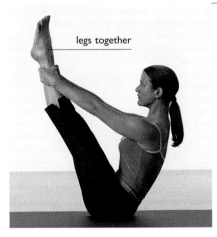

legs together

3 Close the legs, keeping them straight. Open them once again and then bend the knees to return to the Step 1 position. Repeat entire sequence 2–3 times. TRANSITION: *Continue on to the Open Leg Rocker* (see pp82–83) *or lower yourself down to the mat and extend both legs up to 90° for the Corkscrew* (see pp84–85).

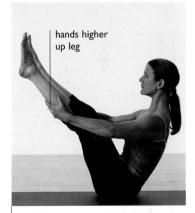

hands higher up leg

MODIFIED HAND POSITION
You may find it necessary to keep your knees slightly bent. If you have trouble maintaining your balance, try placing your hands higher up your legs, towards the calves.

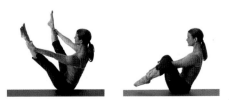

Exhale..........................Rest

OPEN LEG ROCKER

This exercise will challenge your balance, flexibility, and strength. Focus on maintaining a constant shape as you rock. If at first you cannot roll completely up, walk your hands up higher towards the calves. If this still proves too difficult, continue to work on the Open Leg Rocker Preparation (*pp80–81*).

REPETITIONS 5–8 times (Steps 2–4).

CAUTION Avoid this exercise if you have an acute back injury. If you have a sensitive tailbone, proceed with caution.

VISUALIZATION Imagine rolling your spine against the floor in the way that a wheel rolls smoothly back and forth.

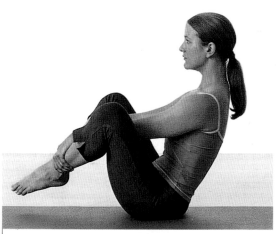

1 Leaving the knees open, bring both feet in towards your buttocks and gently grasp the ankles. Tilt back slightly, until the feet come off the floor, and find your balance.

legs hip width apart

2 Holding the ankles, extend both legs up, hip width apart. Maintain your balance by scooping the abdominals in towards the spine. Keep your chest lifted and your gaze high.

At a glance

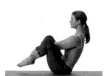

Breathe naturally.....................Inhale to roll back.................Exhale to roll up

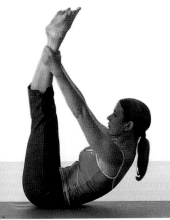

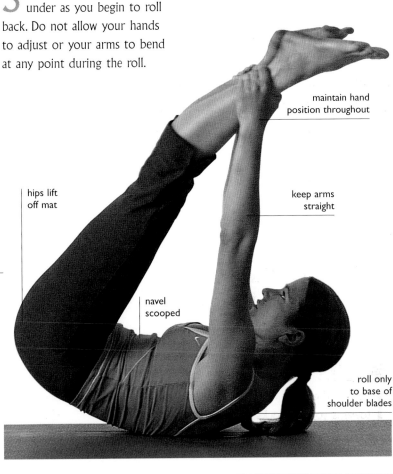

3 Inhale and curl the tail under as you begin to roll back. Do not allow your hands to adjust or your arms to bend at any point during the roll.

maintain hand position throughout

hips lift off mat

keep arms straight

navel scooped

roll only to base of shoulder blades

4 Continue to roll to the base of the shoulder blades. Exhale and reverse the roll to return to your balance point (Step 2). Continue to rock, repeating Steps 2–4, then return to Step 1 to finish.
TRANSITION: *Place your feet flat and lower your body down to the mat, bringing the knees in to the chest to prepare for the Corkscrew* (see pp84–85).

HEAD-TO-TOE CHECKLIST

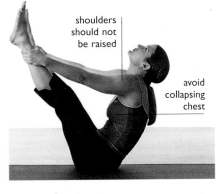

shoulders should not be raised

avoid collapsing chest

• **Do not** initiate with the head.
• **Keep** your rhythm – do not stall or linger at the bottom of the roll.
• **Avoid** "whipping" up. Roll up smoothly with strength and control.
• **Never** roll onto your neck, but only to the base of the shoulder blades.

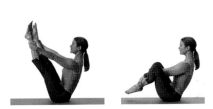

. . . . Rest

CORKSCREW

With your upper body flat on the mat and your legs pivoting above you, the Corkscrew targets the lower part of the abdominals. Move fluidly, avoiding muscle tension or gripping in the upper body or thigh muscles. Begin with small circles and increase their size as your stabilization improves.

REPETITIONS 2–3 sets, alternating direction of circles.

CAUTION For a delicate back, place your hands as shown on p77. For a recent back injury or hernia, omit this exercise.

VISUALIZATION Envision your midsection wrapped tightly in a corset. As your legs circle down away from you, the corset tightens, shrinking your waistline.

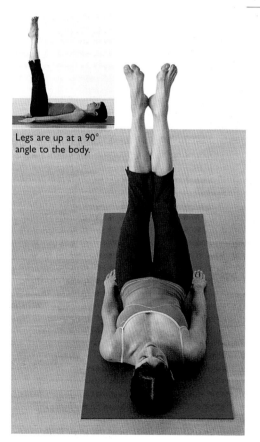

Legs are up at a 90° angle to the body.

1 Lie flat on the mat with both legs up towards the ceiling in Pilates stance. Pin the shoulders back, pressing the backs of the arms and the palms flat into the mat as you lengthen the neck.

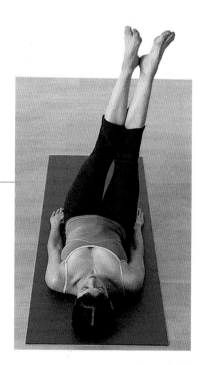

2 Inhale and squeeze your legs together as you carry them to your right side. Do not allow the left side of your body to lift off the mat.

At a glance

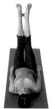 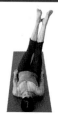 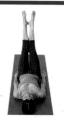 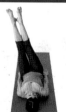 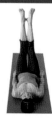

Inhale to circle down.....................Exhale to circle up and reverse

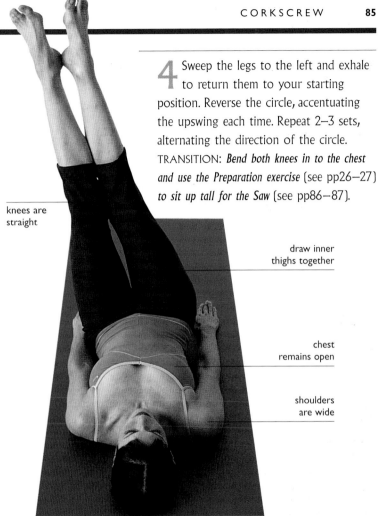

4 Sweep the legs to the left and exhale to return them to your starting position. Reverse the circle, accentuating the upswing each time. Repeat 2–3 sets, alternating the direction of the circle.
TRANSITION: *Bend both knees in to the chest and use the Preparation exercise* (see pp26–27) *to sit up tall for the Saw* (see pp86–87).

knees are straight

draw inner thighs together

chest remains open

shoulders are wide

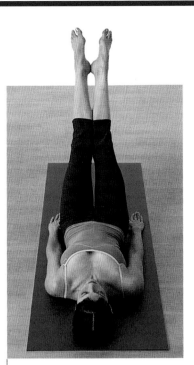

3 Circle the legs down through the centre line of the body. Keep pulling the navel in towards the spine.

HEAD-TO-TOE CHECKLIST

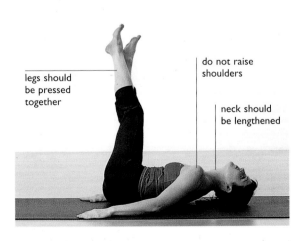

legs should be pressed together

do not raise shoulders

neck should be lengthened

• **Use** your wings to control the upper body as you circle the legs.
• **As you lift t**he legs back up, the lower back remains against the mat. Do not allow the momentum of your legs to lift your hips up.
• **In Step 3**, lower your legs only to your point of control – the abdominals

should never distend.
• **Circle** energetically, sweeping the legs around with dynamic and flow.
• **To advance** the exercise, you may lift the hips on the upswing of each circle, elevating the hips slightly each time. Be sure to lower down with perfect control as you begin to the other side.

SAW

The Saw stretches the body in a rotated position. Your waistline works in opposition to your body as you reach forward to "saw" off your little toe. Remember never to bounce while stretching. To increase flexibility, simply hold your position and breathe deeply, emptying the lungs as you elongate the muscles.

REPETITIONS 2–3 sets (Steps 1–3).

CAUTION Omit this exercise if you have had a recent back injury. If the stretch is too intense in the back of the knees, soften your legs.

VISUALIZATION Imagine being submerged to your hipbones in a bed of sand. Your lower body is immobilized as you reach towards the little toe.

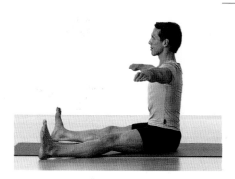

1 Sit tall, reaching your arms out to either side, within your peripheral vision. Open the legs just past the width of your hips and flex the feet.

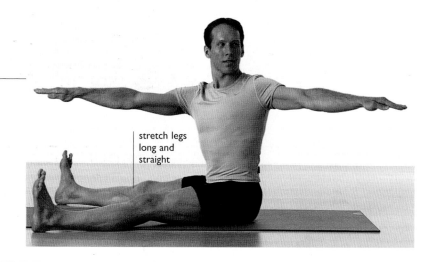

stretch legs long and straight

2 Inhale and twist your waist, carrying the arms with you. Do not adjust your hips but keep the feet and legs stationary. As you twist, the spine lengthens and the chest lifts high.

At a glance

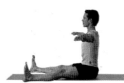
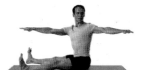
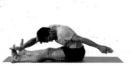
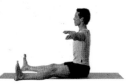

Inhale to sit tall............................Exhale to stretch forward...............Repeat

3 Exhale and round forwards, aiming your little finger to the outside of your little toe. Pull back in the opposite hip as your body reaches forwards, stretching for 3 counts. Inhale and sit tall to begin the exercise to the other side. Alternate sides for 2–3 sets.

TRANSITION: *Flip over on to your stomach for the Advanced Swan Dive* (see pp120–121) *and/or the Intermediate Neck Roll* (see pp88–89).

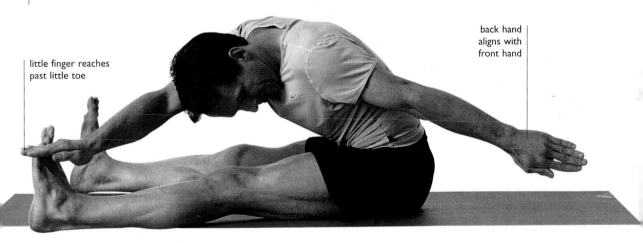

back hand aligns with front hand

little finger reaches past little toe

HEAD-TO-TOE CHECKLIST

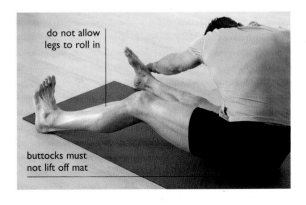

do not allow legs to roll in

buttocks must not lift off mat

• **Twist** above the waist, keeping your sit-bones anchored to the floor.

• **Control** your arms as you twist. Swinging the arms back can strain the shoulders.

• **The back arm** sweeps back and down to line up with the front hand.

• **Hang your head** down and look towards your back hand.

• **Keep** knees and toes pointing to the ceiling.

• **Roll up** through the spine to sit tall before repeating to the other side. Do not come up with a flat back.

NECK ROLL

Having developed enough abdominal strength to perform exercises on the stomach, we now introduce the Neck Roll, in which upper back strength and neck mobility are addressed. The abdominals get to stretch in this position but they must still work to protect the back. Begin small, increasing the arc as you feel more comfortable.

REPETITIONS 1–2 neck rolls in each direction – clockwise and anti-clockwise.

CAUTION Use the modification shown opposite if you experience any shoulder, wrist, or low back strain during this exercise.

VISUALIZATION Envision your body floating up effortlessly like a cobra snaking up into the air.

shoulders pressing down   abdominals lifted   legs pressed together

1 Begin face down on the mat. Place the hands directly under the shoulders and press the arms close to the body. Squeeze the legs tightly together.

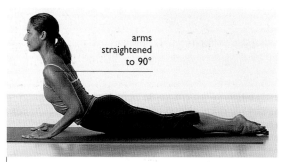

arms straightened to 90°

2 Using little to no hand support, lift your head and upper back slightly. Press the hands firmly into the mat and continue to arc up. Straighten the arms, first to 90° and then as much as possible.

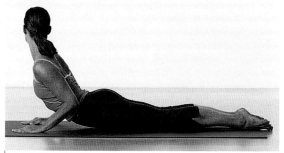

3 Continue to lift your abdominals and press your legs together as you turn your head over one shoulder and gently stretch the neck. Do not twist the shoulders or hips. Do not disrupt your alignment. The shoulders and hips remain square, preserving your box.

At a glance

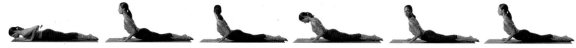

Inhale...............Exhale................Breathe naturally..........Repeat to other side

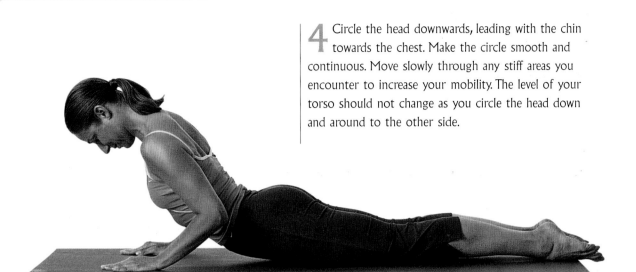

4 Circle the head downwards, leading with the chin towards the chest. Make the circle smooth and continuous. Move slowly through any stiff areas you encounter to increase your mobility. The level of your torso should not change as you circle the head down and around to the other side.

5 Stretch your neck to this side and return to centre, looking straight ahead. Repeat, beginning on the other side.
TRANSITION: *Lower down to the mat for the Advanced Swan Dive* (see pp120–121) *or support yourself on your elbows to prepare for Intermediate Single Leg Kick* (see pp 90–91).

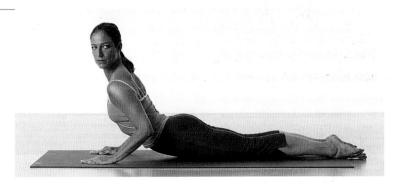

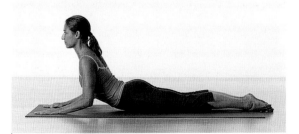

MODIFIED ARM POSITION
If you develop any shoulder, elbow, or wrist pain, simply slide the arms forwards to alleviate the stress on these joints. This modification can also be used to relieve lower back pain should you experience this during the exercise.

HEAD-TO-TOE CHECKLIST

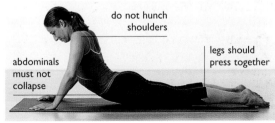

do not hunch shoulders

legs should press together

abdominals must not collapse

• **Lengthen** the back of the neck and the front of the throat.
• **Activate** your wings to keep the shoulders down, away from your ears.

• **Pull** the belly button up towards the spine. Never let the abdominals sag.
• **Keep** the buttocks firm and the legs and heels pressed together.

SINGLE LEG KICK

The Single Leg Kick will strengthen the back of the legs while stretching the front of the hips. The position of the upper body also improves tone in the arms and the muscles of the chest. To gain the most benefit from this exercise, you will need to draw upon a certain amount of coordination and speed.

1 With your fists together, press your forearms into the mat. Lift the sternum and pull the navel up. Wrap the backs of the legs firmly together and pull your shoulder blades down and back.

REPETITIONS 4–5 sets of alternating legs.

CAUTION If the kicking motion brings on knee pain or cramps in the hamstrings, reduce the range of motion and work more slowly.

VISUALIZATION Envision your legs swishing past each other, kicking in time to your heartbeat.

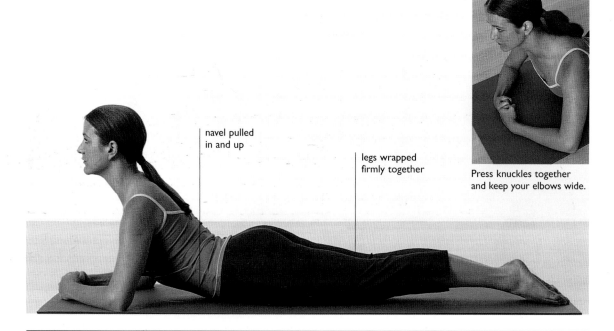

navel pulled in and up

legs wrapped firmly together

Press knuckles together and keep your elbows wide.

At a glance

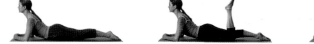 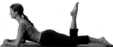 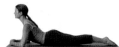

Inhale for one set...................Exhale for next set...............................Rest

2 Kick one leg into your rear end with a quick, double beat. Tighten the buttocks, pressing the front of the hips into the mat. Switch legs and repeat for 4–5 sets, inhaling for one set and exhaling for the next. Return to Step 1 position to finish.
TRANSITION: *Lower one cheek onto the mat and clasp your hands behind your back to prepare for the Double Leg Kick* (see pp92–93).

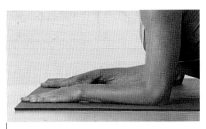

MODIFIED HAND POSITION

If you find it uncomfortable to hold your wrists with the fists together, slide the arms into parallel position with the palms flat on the mat.

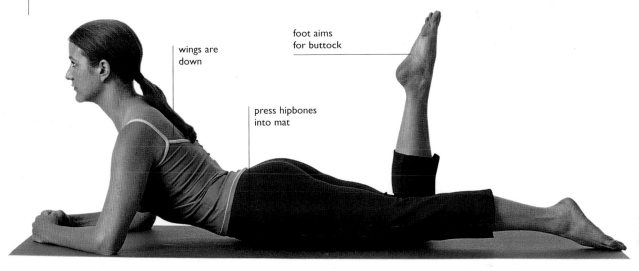

wings are down

foot aims for buttock

press hipbones into mat

HEAD-TO-TOE CHECKLIST

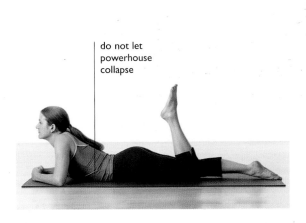

do not let powerhouse collapse

• **Stretch** the back of the neck long and focus the eyes straight ahead.
• **Use** your arms: pressing your arms into the floor will help to lift your body higher.
• **Support** your power-house. Do not let your stomach drop to the mat, collapsing your lower back.

• **Press** the inner thighs together and kick the legs with control.
• **Try to work** the legs just above the mat. As they pass each other in the air, they should immediately rebound back up without touching the floor.

DOUBLE LEG KICK

This exercise helps to increase the mobility of the spine and open the front of the chest. To optimize the motion, modulate your movements and your tempo – move slowly and precisely enough to feel your muscles working, but keep your energy high and your rhythm constant.

REPETITIONS 2–3 sets (Steps 2–4).

CAUTION Avoid this exercise if you have injured your shoulders or collarbones. Use discretion if you have suffered a wrist or back injury.

VISUALIZATION Imagine your final pose as a ship's figurehead. As the ship speeds through the water your body floats higher.

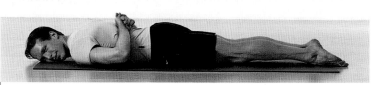

1 Lie face down with your hands clasped behind your back, one cupped inside the other. The palms are face up and the elbows are down. One cheek is on the mat.

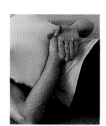

Cup hands as high as possible and press elbows to the mat.

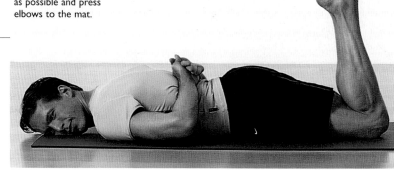

2 Inhale and bend both knees, kicking them into your buttocks for three swift pulses. Keep your hipbones pressed firmly into the mat.

At a glance

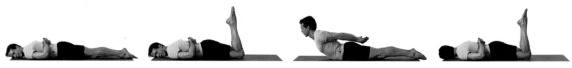

Inhale to kick.....................Exhale to stretch up..............................Repeat

3 Exhale and simultaneously straighten the arms and legs, lifting the upper body up high off the mat. The head is up with the eyes looking straight ahead. The hands reach just above the rear end and the legs stretch right down to the mat.

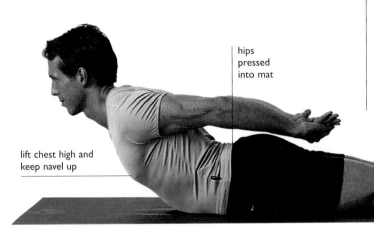

hips pressed into mat

lift chest high and keep navel up

4 Lower the body and turn the head so the other cheek is on the mat. Bring the hands back to their starting position with the elbows down and repeat Steps 2–4 on this side. Perform 2–3 sets, alternating sides.

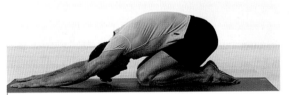

5 Sit back on your heels, in child's pose, to release your lower back. Keep your head down and your arms forwards, but continue to support the abdominals.

TRANSITION: *Roll up to a kneeling position and flip over on to your back for the Neck Pull (see pp94–95).*

HEAD-TO-TOE CHECKLIST

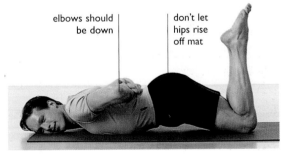

elbows should be down

don't let hips rise off mat

- **Your head** is the highest point as you arc up. Keep the feet firmly on the floor and the hands close to the body.
- **The elbows** and shoulders sink down to the mat when lying flat. If this is impossible, try lowering your hands to the small of the back.
- **Flatten** your hipbones into the mat when kicking the legs.
- **Press** your body up smoothly. Resist any sudden or jerking movements.

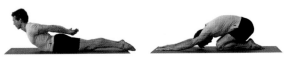

Exhale......................................Rest

NECK PULL

The Neck Pull is a new spin on an old "crunch". Here you will test your ability to work your abdominals in shortened as well as lengthened positions. Spinal articulation and fluidity are the key – the entire sequence is one continuous motion. If you need extra assistance, anchor your feet under a piece of furniture.

REPETITIONS Repeat entire sequence 5–8 times.

CAUTION If you have a stiff spine or have difficulty articulating through the spine, apply one of the modifications shown on p97.

VISUALIZATION Imagine yourself as a marionette. As you lengthen back, the strings attached to your elbows pull upwards, lifting your spine tall and long.

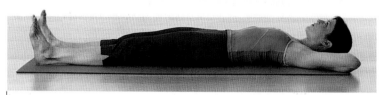

1 Begin lying flat on the mat with your hands layered behind your head and your elbows wide. The legs are hip width apart and the feet are flexed.

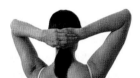

Place one hand over the other at the base of the skull.

2 Inhale as you begin curling forwards. Draw the weight of your head forwards and round up sequentially – head, shoulders, ribs, and finally the pelvis. Pull your waistline in deeply on the way up.

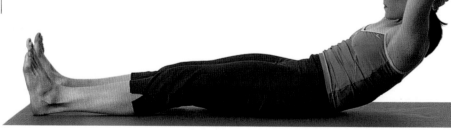

At a glance

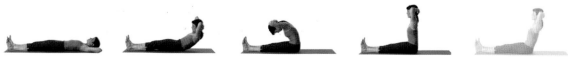

Inhale to curl up.........Exhale to round over........Inhale to sit up and hinge back

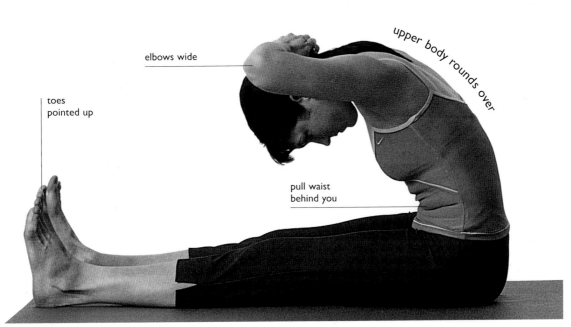

elbows wide

toes
pointed up

upper body rounds over

pull waist
behind you

3 Exhale as your upper body folds over the legs. Do not flatten your back or hinge forwards at the hips. Instead, keep pulling the navel in, scooping out the abdominals. Press the heels forwards to stretch the backs of the legs. The elbows remain lifted.

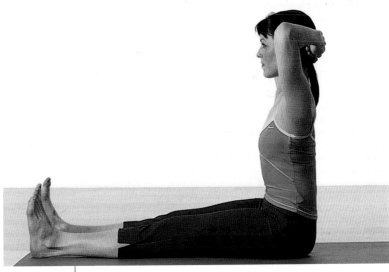

4 Inhale to roll up to a tall, sitting posture, rounding up through each vertebra. Align your head, neck, and spine and lengthen through the sides of the waist. Anchor your heels firmly into the mat and feel the base of your skull pressing firmly into the palms of your hands.

Exhale to lower down......Repeat

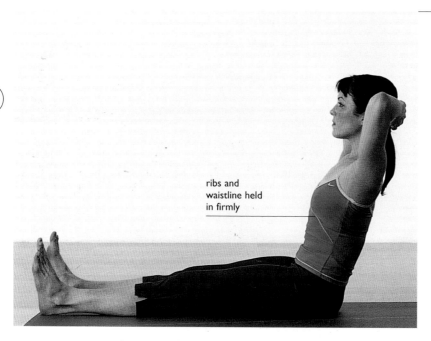

ribs and
waistline held
in firmly

5 Squeeze your bottom and tilt back in a flat line, holding the power-house strong. Exhale as you lean back, keeping your elbows wide and your legs firmly on the mat. The ribs pull in to keep the abdominals flat.

6 Continue to hinge back as far as you can without allowing the stomach muscles to protrude. Begin pressing your back into the mat, curling down vertebra by vertebra. Repeat 5–8 times. Return to Step 1 position to repeat.
TRANSITION: *Lower your arms to your sides for the Advanced Scissors* (see pp122–123) *or roll onto your side for the Intermediate Side Kicks Series* (see pp98–105).

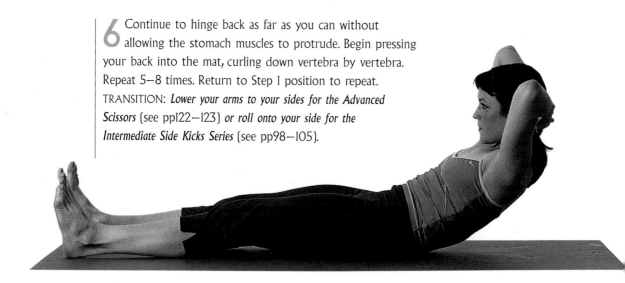

At a glance

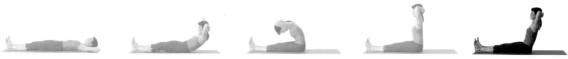

Inhale to curl up.........Exhale to round over.......Inhale to sit up and hinge back

MODIFIED HAND POSITION: 1

To keep your abdominals from bulging out, crawl your hands up your legs as you round up. Keep the knees soft and the heels pressed into the mat.

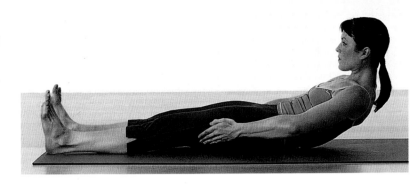

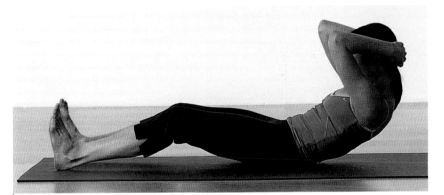

MODIFIED HAND POSITION: 2

If the first modification is too easy, try folding your arms in around your head. You may also combine the two modifications, walking your hands up your legs as you round up and placing them behind your head to lower down.

HEAD-TO-TOE CHECKLIST

do not let legs rise off mat

avoid letting abdominals bulge out

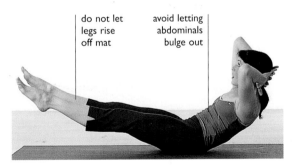

• **Use control**, not momentum. To gain the most strength, slow down through the difficult spots.
• **Remember** – your abdominals attach to your ribs. If you keep your ribs in, you are also keeping your stomach in.
• **Never** tug on your neck. Your powerhouse does the work, not your arms.

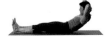 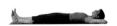

Exhale to lower down......Repeat

SIDE KICKS: PREPARATION

To prepare the body for the lengthy Side Kicks Series, proper set up is critical: stability is provided by correct placement. In side lying, hips and shoulders are aligned above each other. Each exercise in the series moves from the starting position shown below. Perform the entire series to one side before switching to the other leg.

REPETITIONS I only.
Note: The entire Side Kicks Series is performed to one side before switching to the other leg.

CAUTION If resting your head on your hand causes shoulder or arm pain, use the modified position.

VISUALIZATION Imagine a mirror on the ceiling. In the final position, your body should look like a boomerang if seen from above.

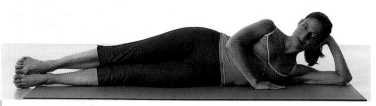

1 Lie on your side and align your body against the back edge of the mat. Prop your head up on one hand and place the palm of the other hand firmly on the mat in front of you.

2 Breathe in, engage your powerhouse, and lift both legs up in one motion. Be sure to work the legs in Pilates stance. Press the shoulders down and relax the neck.

legs in Pilates stance

hip over hip

shoulder over shoulder

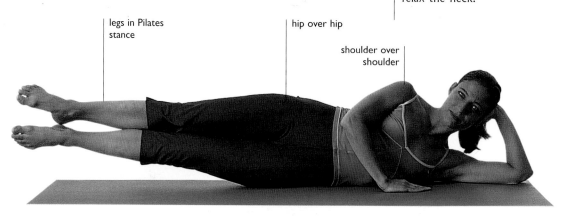

At a glance

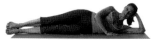 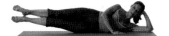 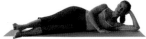

Breathe naturally.........................Inhale...Exhale

3 Exhale as you carry the legs forwards to a 45° angle in front of your body. Place them down on the mat without allowing your hips to slide forwards.

TRANSITION: *You are now ready to move on to the rest of the Side Kicks Series. Begin with the Side Kicks: Front* (see pp100–101).

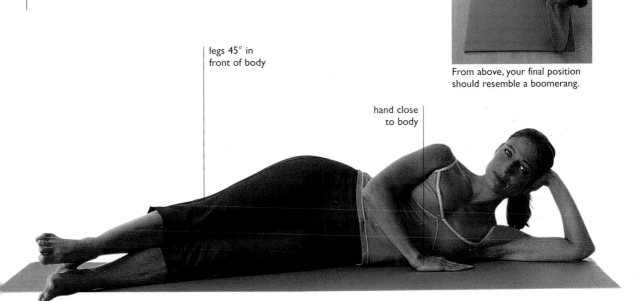

legs 45° in front of body

hand close to body

From above, your final position should resemble a boomerang.

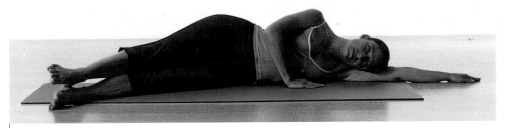

MODIFIED HEAD AND ARM POSITION

If you experience pain or discomfort in your shoulder or wrist, simply extend your arm and lower your head. You may also use a small cushion or a rolled-up towel under your neck for added support.

SIDE KICKS: FRONT

Having established a solid working position, this exercise will challenge your balance in a completely new way. It will stretch the backs of the legs and tone the buttocks. Kick the top leg freely with large, sweeping movements, all the while stabilizing your torso. Hold on to your box and maintain your alignment.

REPETITIONS 5–10 sets (Steps 2–3). *Note: The entire Side Kicks Series is performed to one side before switching to the other leg.*

CAUTION If you experience any neck, shoulder, or wrist pain, extend your lower arm along the mat and rest your head (see p99).

VISUALIZATION Imagine your leg swinging like the pendulum of a clock while the body holds still.

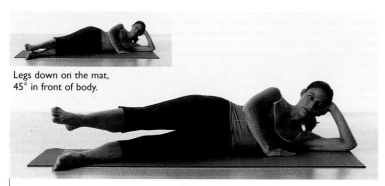

Legs down on the mat, 45° in front of body.

1 From the final Preparation position (*see pp98–99*) elevate your top leg just in line with your hip. Rotate the leg into Pilates stance.

2 Inhale and swing the upper leg forwards for a double pulse. Keep the chest high and shoulders and hips stacked above each other. Keep the top leg directly in line with the hip, parallel to the floor.

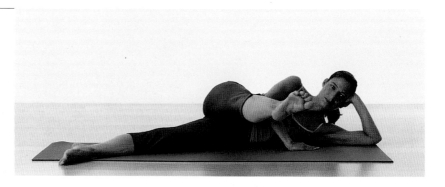

At a glance

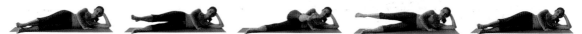

Inhale to kick front.................Exhale to kick back................................Rest

3 Now exhale and swing the leg back, stretching the front of the hip. Firm the rear end, paying special attention to the crease where the back of the leg meets the buttocks. Repeat 5–10 times. To finish, rest the top leg on the bottom leg.

TRANSITION: *Move directly on to the Side Kicks: Up/Down* (see pp102–103).

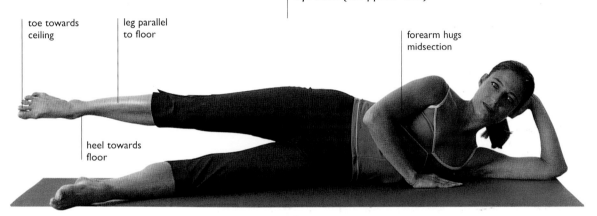

toe towards ceiling

leg parallel to floor

forearm hugs midsection

heel towards floor

MODIFIED HEAD AND ARM POSITIONS

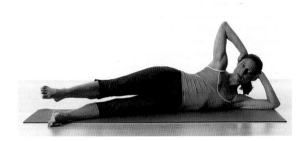

To advance the exercise, perform 5 sets with the hand on the mat and 5 sets with the hand behind the head. Point the elbow to the ceiling and hold it still as you work the legs. The entire Side Kicks Series may be performed in this way.

HEAD-TO-TOE CHECKLIST

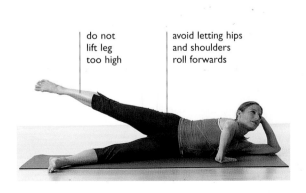

do not lift leg too high

avoid letting hips and shoulders roll forwards

- **Maintain** your elbow at the back edge of the mat.
- **Keep** the neck and shoulders relaxed and the head looking straight out.
- **Don't** let the shoulders roll forwards or back as you kick your leg.
- **Your hand** on the mat is close to the body, with the forearm pressed into your midsection.
- **Pull** the lower abdominals in and up as though you had zipped up a tight pair of trousers.
- **Avoid** any change in the rotation or the height of the leg as it swings to the back.

SIDE KICKS: UP/DOWN

We progress the Side Kicks Series by moving the work of the leg from front to side. Do not disrupt your starting placement – even large, fast movements such as this require total muscle authority. Concentrate on lengthening out: by the end of this exercise, your kicking leg should feel longer than the other one.

REPETITIONS 5–10 times. *Note: Perform the entire Side Kicks Series to one side before switching to other leg.*

CAUTION Modify the exercise by extending your bottom arm as in the Side Kicks: Preparation (*see pp98–99*).

VISUALIZATION Envision your kicking leg as the handle of a water pump. Although it glides up easily, it requires pressure to lower down.

1 Begin as you did in the Side Kicks: Front (*see pp100–101*). The legs are at a 45° angle and the head rests on the hand. The hand on the mat rests close to the body with the forearm pressed against the torso and the palm flat on the mat.

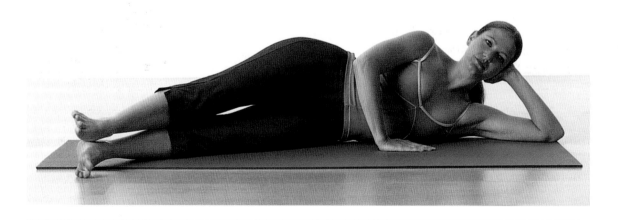

At a glance

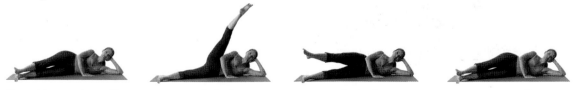

Breathe naturally.............Inhale.................Exhale.........................Repeat

2 Rotate your top leg so that the kneecap and the top of the foot face the ceiling. Inhale and kick the leg up without changing your hips. Keep your head in line with your spine as you kick, resisting any temptation to collapse the chest.

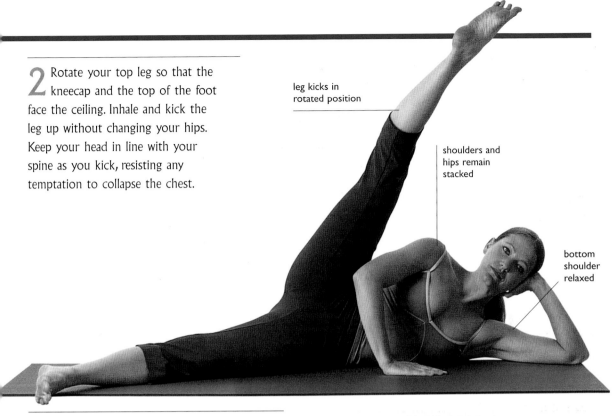

leg kicks in rotated position

shoulders and hips remain stacked

bottom shoulder relaxed

3 Exhale and slowly lower the leg with resistance. Aim the top heel just past the bottom heel. Reach the leg as long as possible, lengthening your waist. Repeat 5–10 times. For an additional challenge, place the hand on the mat behind the head for the last 5 kicks. TRANSITION: *Move directly on to the Side Kicks: Circles (see pp104–105).*

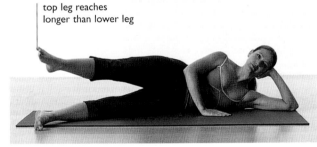

top leg reaches longer than lower leg

HEAD-TO-TOE CHECKLIST

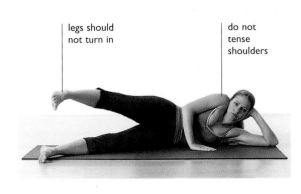

legs should not turn in

do not tense shoulders

• **The neck** and shoulders remain relaxed.

• **Stabilize** the body with the powerhouse. Nothing moves but the kicking leg.

• **Activate** the buttocks to rotate the leg. The heel faces down and the toe faces up.

• **Pay special** attention to the top hip as you kick the leg. Do not allow it to shift back or fall behind the bottom hip.

• **Imagine** yourself from above: the shoulders and hips remain stacked.

• **Stretch the leg** long as you lower it but do not grip the thigh muscles.

SIDE KICKS: CIRCLES

By this time you will have established a secure position to perform the side-lying series. The Side Kicks: Circles are smaller and faster than the previous two exercises and will help to increase the speed and agility with which you can move. Concentrate on isolating the leg in the hip socket and holding the body still and controlled.

REPETITIONS 5–8 circles in each direction, clockwise and anti-clockwise. *Note: The entire Side Kicks Series is performed to one side before switching to the other leg.*

CAUTION If you experience any neck, shoulder, or wrist pain, adopt the modification shown on p99.

VISUALIZATION Move continuously as if you had a tiny hula hoop looped around your ankle.

1 Begin as you did for the Side Kicks: Up/Down *(see pp102–103)*. The legs remain at a 45° angle and the hand is directly in front of you, placed firmly on the mat.

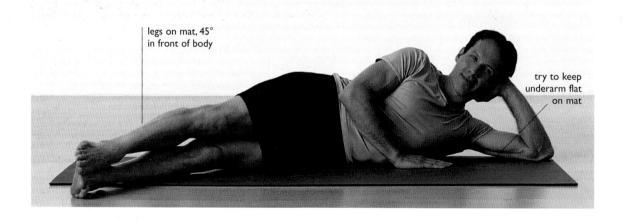

legs on mat, 45° in front of body

try to keep underarm flat on mat

At a glance

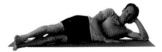
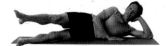
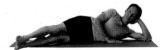

Breathe naturally throughout..Rest

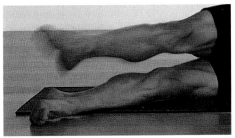

Aim the top heel towards the bottom heel while circling. Keep the thigh muscles loose throughout.

2 Elevate the top leg, just in line with the hip. Begin circling small and swift, brushing the top heel past the bottom heel each time around. Repeat 5–8 times then repeat in the opposite direction. Return to Step 1 position before performing the Side Kicks Series with the other leg. If you wish, perform the Transition: Heel Beats (*pp138–139*) to change position.

TRANSITION: *Remain where you are for the Advanced Side Kicks: Double Leg Lift (see pp132–133) or roll onto your back for the Intermediate Teaser Preparation (see pp106–107).*

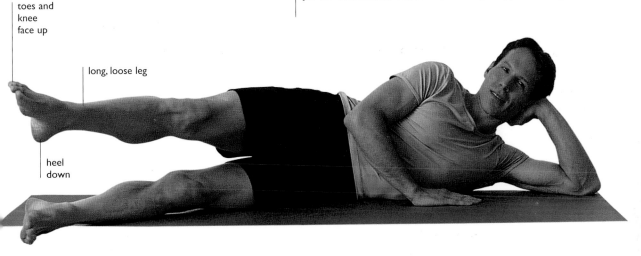

toes and
knee
face up

long, loose leg

heel
down

HEAD-TO-TOE CHECKLIST

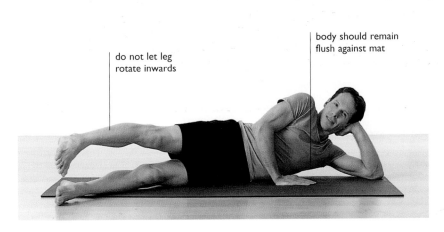

do not let leg
rotate inwards

body should remain
flush against mat

• **Avoid** rising up on your elbow. Try to keep your underarm flat on the mat.

• **Press** the wings down to lengthen the neck.

• **Do not rely** on your hand on the mat: your powerhouse does the work.

• **Work** the top leg in Pilates position without gripping the thigh muscles. Keep a long, loose leg.

TEASER: PREPARATION

Combining strength and power with length and control, the Teaser is the quintessential Pilates exercise. To prepare, we abbreviate the exercise and concentrate on purifying the movement. Our aim is to eliminate all other muscle groups from taking over the work of the powerhouse. Take your time and be precise.

REPETITIONS Repeat entire sequence 2–3 times.

CAUTION If you cannot rise up without bulging the midsection, use your hands to crawl up the sides of your legs. Alternatively, have a partner hold your feet in place.

VISUALIZATION Imagine that someone is gently pulling you forward by the tips of your fingers until you are sitting tall.

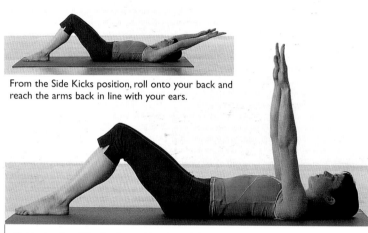

From the Side Kicks position, roll onto your back and reach the arms back in line with your ears.

2 Follow the arm motion by raising your head and shoulders and peeling your spine off the mat. Breathe in and flatten the abdominals, squeezing your inner thighs together as you curl up.

1 Lie back with the knees bent and your legs pressed together. The feet are flat on the mat. With the arms overhead, keep your back on the mat and your rib cage relaxed. Smoothly raise the arms up in line with your eyes.

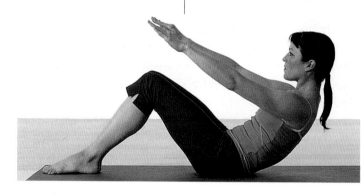

At a glance

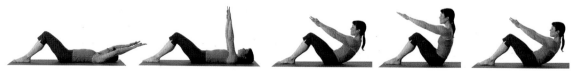

Inhale..Exhale........................Inhale

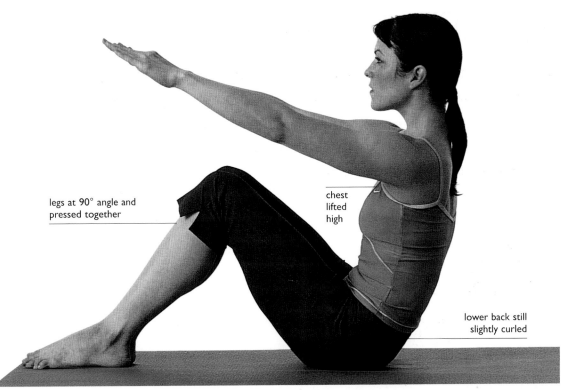

legs at 90° angle and
pressed together

chest
lifted
high

lower back still
slightly curled

3 Exhale and continue rolling up, articulating
through the spine. Reach the arms just above
the knees. Sit upright but stay just behind your
sit-bones so that the abdominals continue to work.
Slowly lower down, pressing one vertebra at a time
into the mat, and return to your starting position
with the arms overhead. Repeat 2–3 times.
TRANSITION: *Draw the knees in to ready yourself for
Teaser 1 (see pp108–109). If you have mastered the
Teaser Preparation, you may skip it and begin the Teaser
Series with Teaser 1.*

HEAD-TO-TOE CHECKLIST

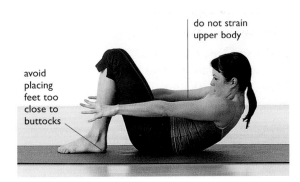

do not strain
upper body

avoid
placing
feet too
close to
buttocks

- **Engage** your wings – the
neck and shoulders should
not work to lift you up.
- **Hold** your ribs in when
reaching the arms over-
head. Do not allow your
back to arch off the mat.

- **Adjust** feet as necessary.
Placing the feet further
away from the buttocks
makes it easier to sit up,
and vice versa.
- **Go** slowly – do not rely
on momentum.

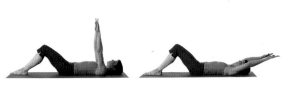

Exhale................................Repeat

TEASER 1

Humorously referred to as the "mother of all sit-ups", this exercise effectively eliminates muscle substitution or cheating and allows the purest possible access to your core muscles. At the peak of the exercise, momentarily hold the position, "teasing" the balance.

REPETITIONS 1–2 sets (each set with 3 repetitions of Steps 2–4).

CAUTION If you suffer from a stiff spine, practise the Teaser Preparation, or perform the exercise with your feet against a wall.

VISUALIZATION As you roll down, imagine each vertebra arriving on the mat the way your fingers might travel down the keys of a piano.

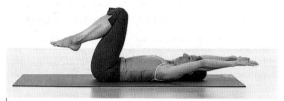

1 Begin lying on your back, with your knees drawn in and your arms overhead, by your ears. Do not allow your back to arch or your ribs to protrude.

2 Extend both legs up to a 45° angle and rotate into Pilates stance. The legs are long and straight but not locked. Maintain your scoop and keep the back towards the mat. Inhale to prepare without distending the ribs.

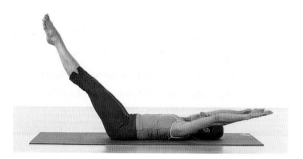

At a glance

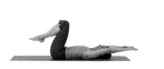 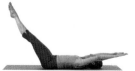 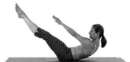 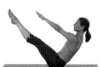

Inhale..Exhale

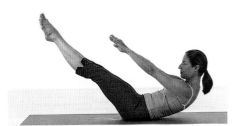

3 Raise your arms, your head, and your shoulders in sequence, curling the body up off the mat vertebra by vertebra. The chin is towards the chest and the fingers reach for the toes. Avoid tensing the thigh muscles as you curl higher up; instead, sink the navel deeper.

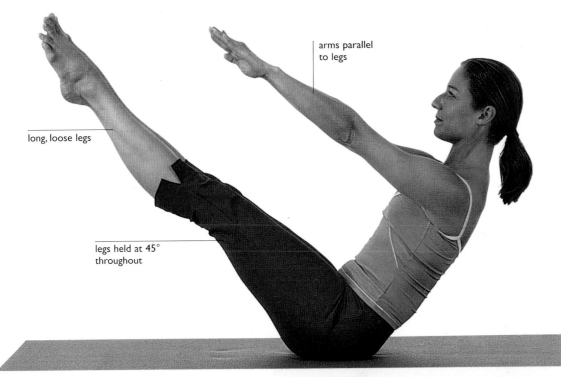

arms parallel to legs

long, loose legs

legs held at 45° throughout

4 Sit up in a "V" shape. Keep your legs up as you slowly lower, one segment at a time. Rise up twice more, rest, and repeat. TRANSITION: *Perform 1 set before the Advanced Teaser 2 (see pp140–141) or perform 2 sets and sit up for the Intermediate Seal (see pp110–111).*

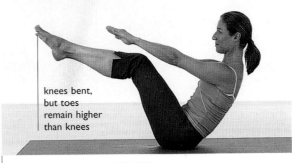

knees bent, but toes remain higher than knees

MODIFIED LEG POSITION
If you have difficulty sitting up all the way, slightly bend the knees, keeping the toes suspended higher than the knees as you lift and lower the body.

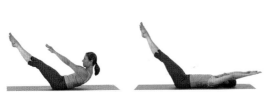

Inhale.................Exhale........Repeat

SEAL

The final exercise in the intermediate program is the Seal, so-called because of Mr Pilates' image of a seal clapping its flippers. Designed to work the entire body in a continuous rolling motion, the Seal tests your balance and coordination. Start at the front edge of your mat so you will have enough room to roll back and forth.

REPETITIONS Repeat entire sequence 5–8 times.

CAUTION Omit this exercise if you have an acute back injury. If you have a delicate wrist or elbow, proceed with caution.

VISUALIZATION Envision your body as a perpetual motion model, rolling back and forth effortlessly.

1 Draw the feet in towards your centre and wrap one hand around the outside of each ankle. Tip back to balance on your tailbone, bringing the feet just above the floor. Keep the knees within your frame and scoop the navel deeper.

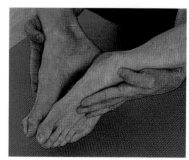

Hands are wrapped around the ankles. Do not let soles of feet come together.

At a glance

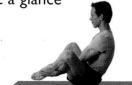
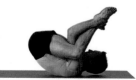
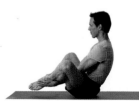

Inhale to roll back..Exhale to roll up.........Repeat

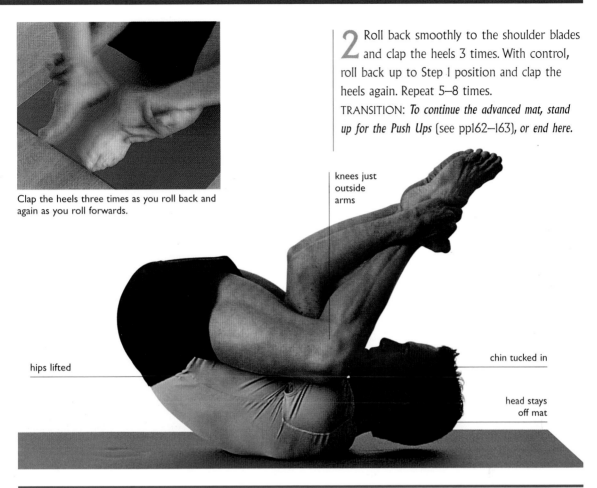

2 Roll back smoothly to the shoulder blades and clap the heels 3 times. With control, roll back up to Step 1 position and clap the heels again. Repeat 5–8 times.

TRANSITION: *To continue the advanced mat, stand up for the Push Ups (see pp162–163), or end here.*

Clap the heels three times as you roll back and again as you roll forwards.

knees just outside arms

chin tucked in

head stays off mat

hips lifted

HEAD-TO-TOE CHECKLIST

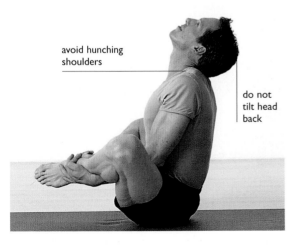

avoid hunching shoulders

do not tilt head back

• **Never** roll onto your head or shoulders – only to the base of the shoulder blades.
• **Initiate** rolling back from the powerhouse, not from the head.
• **Keep** the shoulders relaxed and the chin towards the chest as you roll.
• **Knees** are only shoulder width apart: this keeps the feet in correct alignment.
• **Roll up** slightly slower than you rolled back, to challenge the abdominals.
• **Lift** the hips as you roll back. This will help to massage the spine as you roll back and forth.
• **Avoid momentum** when rolling up. Instead, roll up slightly slower than you rolled back, to challenge the abdominals.

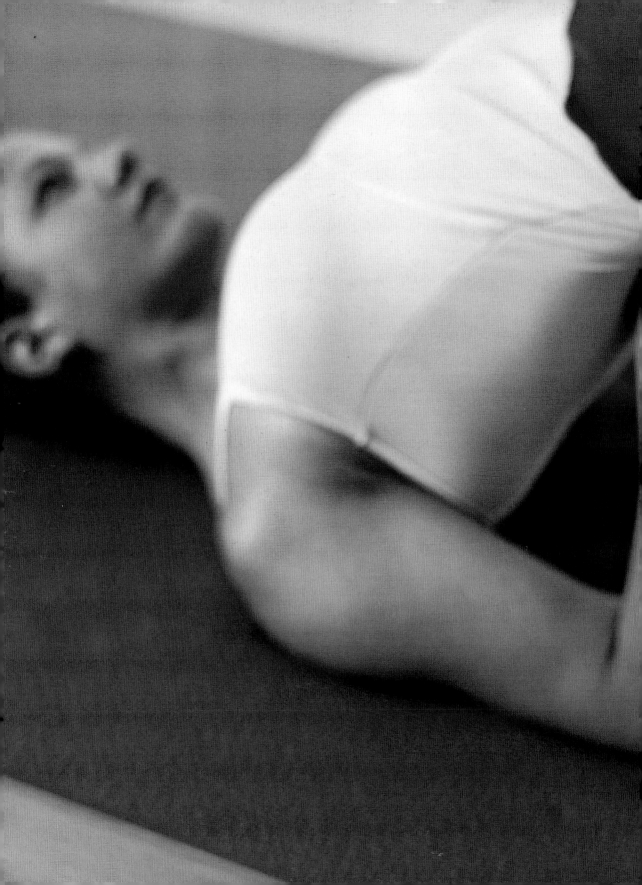

4

ADVANCED PROGRAMME

Each exercise in this section requires a mastery of the earlier material as well as a complete understanding of the fundamental approach to Pilates. Add this final layer of exercises cautiously, choosing only one at a time, and in the order given. While control and precision can always be improved upon, *flow* becomes our goal at this final level.

EXERCISE SEQUENCE

The advanced exercise sequence chart represents the full Pilates mat workout the way
it was originally intended to be performed. It includes many new exercises, which are
integrated with others from earlier programmes. As before, each exercise ends with
transition instructions to help you segue smoothly from one exercise to the next.

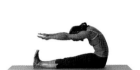

1 The Hundred
(pp48–49)

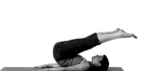

2 Roll Up
(pp50–51)

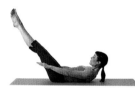

3 Roll Over
(pp116–119)

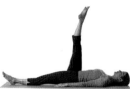

4 Single Leg Circles
(pp52–53)

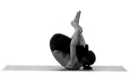

5 Rolling Like a Ball
(pp54–55)

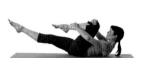

6 Single Leg Stretch
(pp56–57)

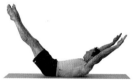

7 Double Leg Stretch
(pp58–59)

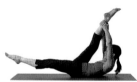

8 Single Straight Leg
Stretch (pp74–75)

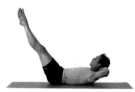

9 Double Straight Leg
Stretch (pp76–77)

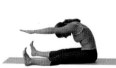

10 Criss-Cross
(pp78–79)

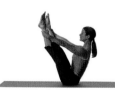

11 Spine Stretch
Forward (pp60–61)

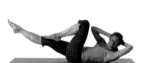

12 Open Leg Rocker
(pp82–83)

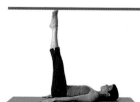

13 Corkscrew
(pp84–85)

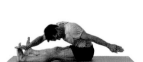

14 Saw
(pp86–87)

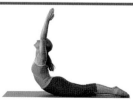

15 Swan Dive
(pp120–121)

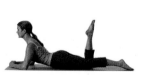

16 Single Leg Kick
(pp90–91)

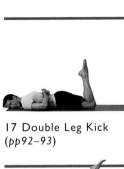

17 Double Leg Kick
(pp92–93)

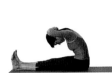

18 Neck Pull
(pp94–97)

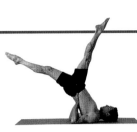

19 Scissors
(pp122–123)

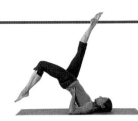

20 Bicycle
(pp124–125)

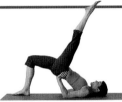

21 Shoulder Bridge
(pp126–127)

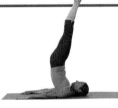

22 Spine Twist
(pp128–129)

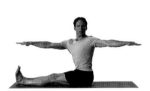

23 Jack Knife
(pp130–131)

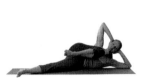

24 Side Kicks Series
(pp98–105; 132–137)

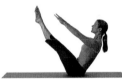

25 Teaser Series
(pp106–109; 140–143)

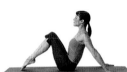

26 Hip Circles
(pp146–147)

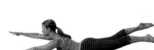

27 Swimming
(pp148–149)

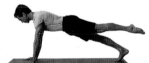

28 Leg Pull Down
(pp150–151)

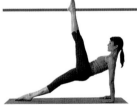

29 Leg Pull Up
(pp152–153)

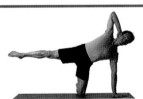

30 Kneeling Side Kicks
(pp154–155)

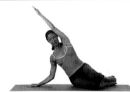

31 Mermaid
(pp156–157)

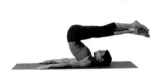

32 Boomerang
(pp158–161)

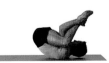

33 Seal
(pp110–111)

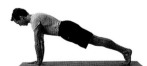

34 Push Ups
(pp162–163)

ROLL OVER

The first advanced level exercise we add is the Roll Over, which, essentially, reverses the Roll Up (*see pp50–51*). Here, we initiate the movement from the bottom of the abdominals rather than from the top. Think of this as a massage to the spine, working each vertebra against the floor.

REPETITIONS 3 times with legs together when lifting, 3 times with legs apart.

CAUTION Omit this exercise if you have a delicate neck or a recent back injury.

VISUALIZATION As you lift overhead, imagine performing this exercise in a low-ceilinged room. Keep your body and legs contained within this small space.

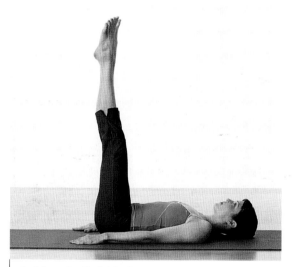

1 After the Roll Up, lower both arms to the mat and draw both legs in and up to a 90° angle, pressing the backs of the legs together. Press your shoulders and palms flat into the mat and anchor the powerhouse firmly.

2 Inhale and initiate from the powerhouse to float your hips up, bringing the legs over your head. Keep reaching the arms long. Do not press up onto your neck.

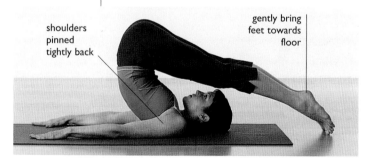

shoulders pinned tightly back

gently bring feet towards floor

At a glance

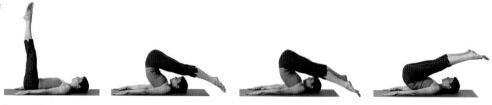

Breathe in to roll over..Breath out to

3 Exhale and separate the legs just past shoulder width. Keep the back of your neck long, avoiding any tensing or crunching in the front of the neck. The arms continue to press firmly into the mat. Your body weight should rest squarely in between your shoulder blades.

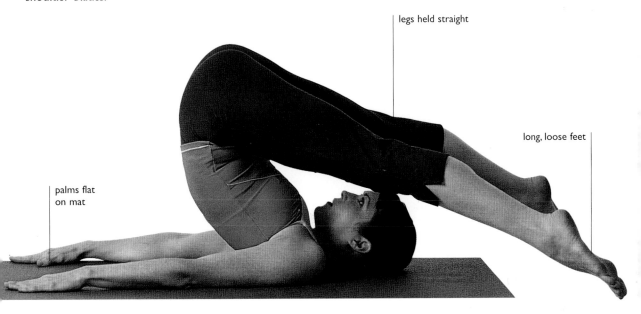

legs held straight

long, loose feet

palms flat on mat

4 Begin rolling back down towards the mat, articulating through the spine until the buttocks reach the mat. The legs follow the spine, pressing close to the body. Descend evenly ensuring that both sides of your back arrive on the mat at the same time. The shoulders should remain relaxed.

legs remain close to body

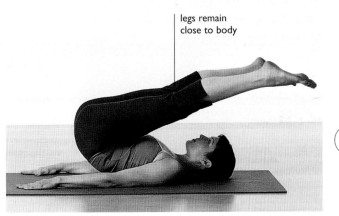

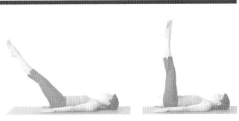

roll down........................Repeat

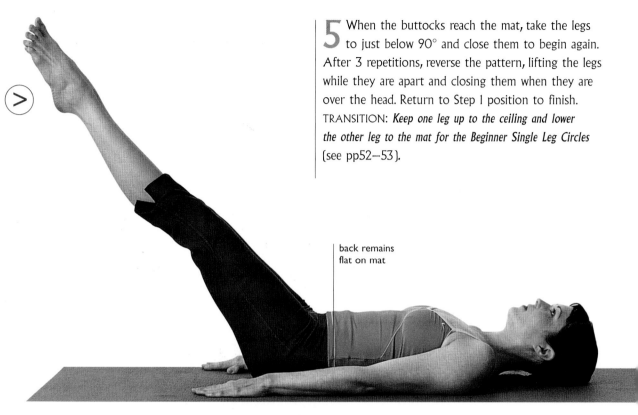

5 When the buttocks reach the mat, take the legs to just below 90° and close them to begin again. After 3 repetitions, reverse the pattern, lifting the legs while they are apart and closing them when they are over the head. Return to Step 1 position to finish.
TRANSITION: *Keep one leg up to the ceiling and lower the other leg to the mat for the Beginner Single Leg Circles* (see pp52–53).

back remains
flat on mat

MODIFIED LEG POSITION

You may work the legs parallel to the floor if you have a stiff back or tight legs. Keep the range of motion smaller, working only to your point of control. Flexible individuals may push the heels back as the legs reach towards the floor, flexing the feet for an added stretch.

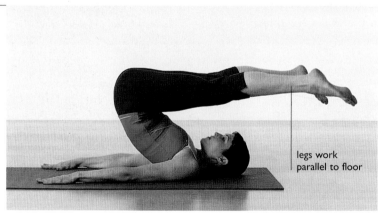

legs work
parallel to floor

At a glance

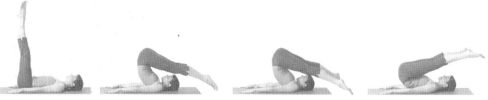

Breathe in to roll over...Breath out to

HEAD-TO-TOE CHECKLIST

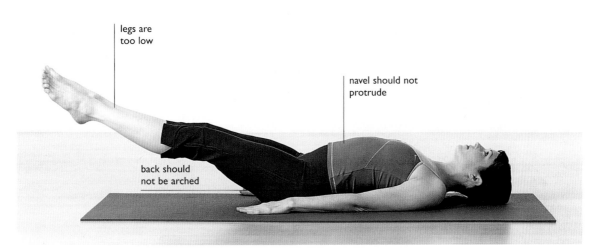

legs are
too low

navel should not
protrude

back should
not be arched

• **Keep** your back flat on the mat as you bring the legs down. If your back arches up off the mat, your legs have gone too low.
• **Anchor** the body into the mat: the shoulders, palms, and powerhouse are all firmly planted into the floor.

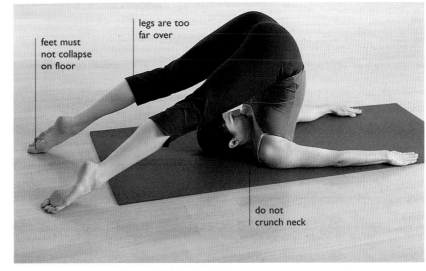

feet must
not collapse
on floor

legs are too
far over

do not
crunch neck

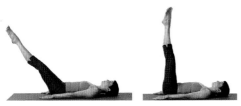

roll down......................Repeat

• **Do not** roll onto your neck. Maintain space between your chin and your chest when the legs are raised over the head.
• **During Step 2**, lift your hips up even before you lift your legs over.
• **Avoid** "swinging" the legs up. Instead, carry them over in a seamless, controlled manner.
• **While** rolling back to the mat, drag the legs close to the chest.
• **Aim** the tips of the toes for the floor, not the tops of the arches.

SWAN DIVE

The Swan Dive is the next progression of the Neck Roll (*see pp88–89*) and is a very advanced exercise. It is one of the few exercises where you will use momentum as well as control and precision. Concentrate on moving the entire body in one solid piece, gradually increasing the range of motion with each repetition.

REPETITIONS 4–6 times (Steps 3–4).

CAUTION Proceed with caution if you have any wrist or shoulder injuries. You may omit this exercise if you have a history of back injury.

VISUALIZATION Imagine your hands and feet are the opposite ends of a seesaw as you dive up and down.

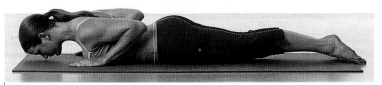

1 Begin face down with your hands under your shoulders and abdominals supported. Lengthen your legs on the mat. Tighten the backs of your thighs and buttocks, pressing them firmly together.

2 Engage the muscles of your upper and middle back to press your body up into a high arc. Straighten your arms as much as possible. If you have done the Neck Roll, continue on to Step 3. If not, lower your body slowly down to the mat and rise up again 2–3 times as a warm-up.

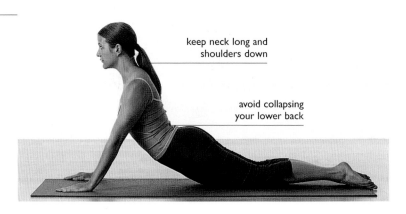

keep neck long and shoulders down

avoid collapsing your lower back

At a glance

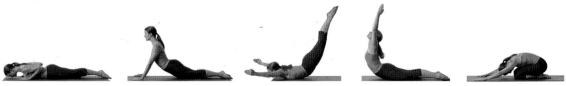

Breathe naturally............................Inhale............Exhale....................Rest

3 Release your hands from the mat and toss your arms out in front of you. Dive forwards like a seesaw, swinging your legs up behind you.

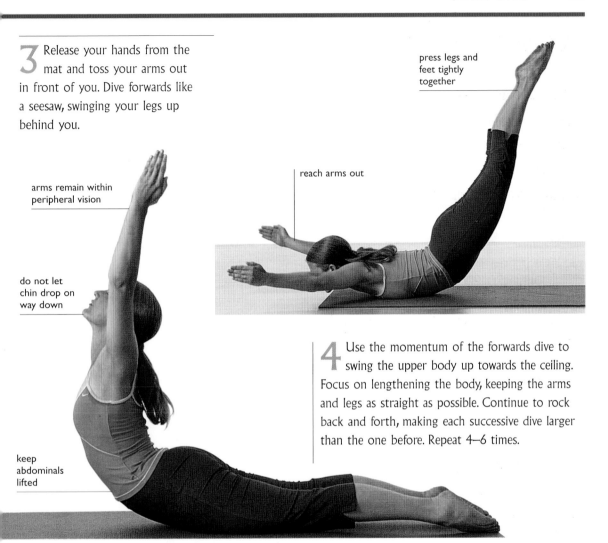

press legs and feet tightly together

reach arms out

arms remain within peripheral vision

do not let chin drop on way down

keep abdominals lifted

4 Use the momentum of the forwards dive to swing the upper body up towards the ceiling. Focus on lengthening the body, keeping the arms and legs as straight as possible. Continue to rock back and forth, making each successive dive larger than the one before. Repeat 4–6 times.

5 After the last repetition, place your hands on the mat and push back onto your heels for a counterstretch. Rest here for several moments to relax the back.
TRANSITION: *Roll up to a kneeling position then extend your body along the mat, propped up on your forearms, for the Intermediate Single Leg Kick (see pp90–91).*

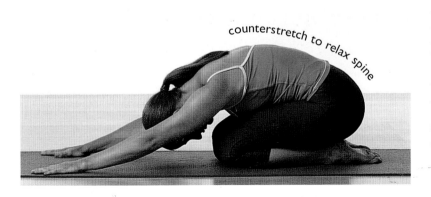

counterstretch to relax spine

SCISSORS

The Scissors challenges your body by shifting your centre of gravity. Here the trunk must hold strong as the legs move freely – not unlike synchronized swimming. Your aim is to open up the front of the hips, which is an area of tightness for most people. The next three exercises can be thought of as the "underwater series".

REPETITIONS 3–4 sets of alternating legs.

CAUTION Use discretion if you have difficulty bearing weight on your shoulders, elbows, or wrists. If you become dizzy, omit the exercise.

VISUALIZATION Imagine you are performing this exercise in a swimming pool, working your legs against the resistance of the water.

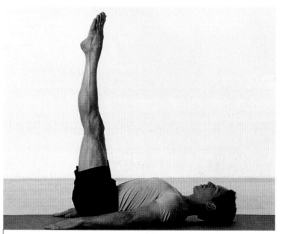

1 Following the Neck Pull (*pp94–97*), lie flat on your back with your legs up to the ceiling. Lengthen the back of your neck and pull your shoulders down and back.

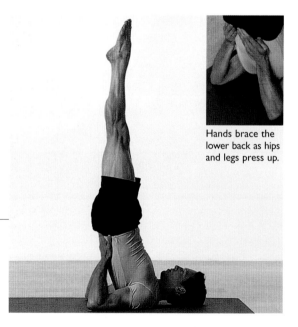

Hands brace the lower back as hips and legs press up.

2 In one fluid motion, press your hips and legs up over your head. Place your hands behind your back. Do not sink your weight into your elbows – keep pressing your hips up.

At a glance

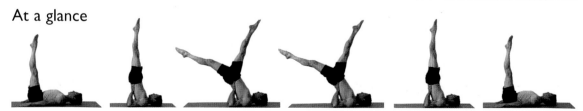

Breathe naturally.............Inhale.............Exhale....................................Rest

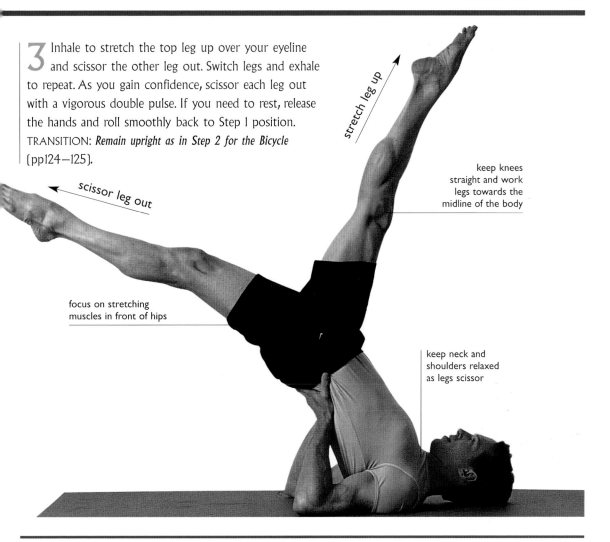

3 Inhale to stretch the top leg up over your eyeline and scissor the other leg out. Switch legs and exhale to repeat. As you gain confidence, scissor each leg out with a vigorous double pulse. If you need to rest, release the hands and roll smoothly back to Step 1 position.
TRANSITION: *Remain upright as in Step 2 for the Bicycle (pp124–125).*

scissor leg out

stretch leg up

keep knees straight and work legs towards the midline of the body

focus on stretching muscles in front of hips

keep neck and shoulders relaxed as legs scissor

HEAD-TO-TOE CHECKLIST

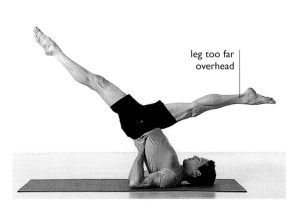

leg too far overhead

• **Lift your hips** in a smooth, controlled manner. You may find you need to slightly adjust your hand position.
• **During Step 3** do not allow the top leg to drop over your head or your legs to open in a split as this will not challenge your centre. Instead, work as though there is a wall just behind your head: do not allow your top leg to touch this imaginary wall.
• **Check that** the legs scissor close together: do not allow the forward-reaching leg to drift or open to the side.
• **Press** the upper arms firmly into the mat.

BICYCLE

The second in the "underwater series", this exercise picks up where the Scissors (*see pp122–123*) left off. We continue to focus on opening the front of the hips by adding a pedaling motion. Pedal slowly to enhance your coordination and agility and gradually increase your range of motion without sacrificing your balance or control.

REPETITIONS 3–4 times in each direction, pedaling forwards and backwards.

CAUTION Use discretion if you have difficulty bearing weight on your shoulders, elbows, or wrists. If you become dizzy during the exercise, roll down and rest.

VISUALIZATION Imagine being underwater. Move continuously against the resistance of the water.

1 From the end of the Scissors, go on to Step 3. Otherwise begin on your back with both legs extended straight up and rotated into Pilates stance. Stretch the back of the neck long and draw the navel in and up.

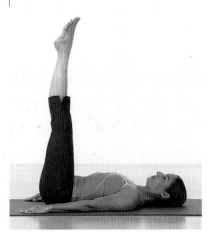

feet remain above eyes

2 In one motion, raise your hips, bringing your legs up directly over your eyes. Place your hands behind your back to help support you (*see p122*). Continue to work the legs in Pilates stance as you progress to Step 3.

At a glance

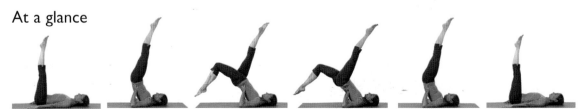

Breathe naturally...................Exhale as each leg pedals out.....................Rest

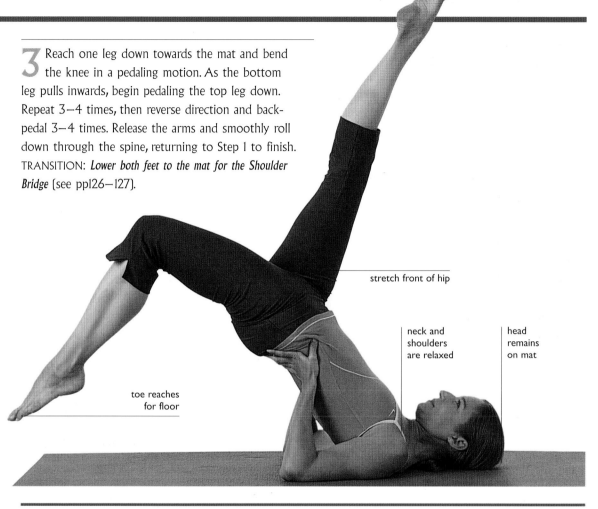

3 Reach one leg down towards the mat and bend the knee in a pedaling motion. As the bottom leg pulls inwards, begin pedaling the top leg down. Repeat 3–4 times, then reverse direction and back-pedal 3–4 times. Release the arms and smoothly roll down through the spine, returning to Step 1 to finish.
TRANSITION: *Lower both feet to the mat for the Shoulder Bridge* (see pp126–127).

stretch front of hip

neck and shoulders are relaxed

head remains on mat

toe reaches for floor

HEAD-TO-TOE CHECKLIST

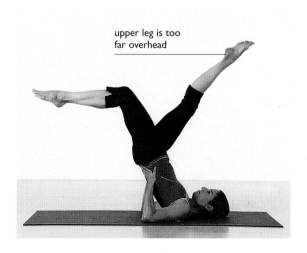

upper leg is too far overhead

• **Hold** your torso solidly in one position. Avoid any twisting motion.
• **Use** the top leg as a counterweight to the pedaling leg. The foot should remain aligned almost perpendicular to the floor.
• **Pedal** each leg as low as possible, bending it only at the deepest point in the stretch. The tip of the toe reaches as close to the floor as possible.
• **Flow** continuously as though you were actually pedaling a bicycle.
• **Draw** the navel in and up to avoid arching the back.
• **Focus** on making each pedal as long as possible. Quick, shortened movements will diminish the benefits of the exercise.

SHOULDER BRIDGE

Our underwater series ends with the Shoulder Bridge. Here, we combine several dynamics; although your control level must remain constant, you will use two distinct tempos throughout the exercise. The pelvis is your power centre for this movement, allowing you to move your legs easily.

REPETITIONS 3 kicks with each leg.

CAUTION Use discretion if you have difficulty bearing weight on your shoulders, elbows, or wrists. If you become dizzy, roll down and rest.

VISUALIZATION Imagine your leg as the hand of a clock. Begin at 9 o'clock and kick towards 2 o'clock with each repetition.

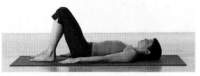

Legs are parallel and hip width apart, knees are bent, and both feet are on the mat.

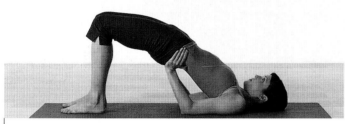

1 Lie on the mat and press up to a "bridge" position. The legs are arranged with the hips, knees, and feet in perfect alignment. Bring your elbows directly into your sides and place your hands under your hips. The thumbs should remain with the rest of the fingers.

2 Straighten one leg, extending it alongside the other. Make sure your hips remain level and your knees are aligned right next to one another. Your body now resembles a plank with your shoulders, hips, and leg all in one line.

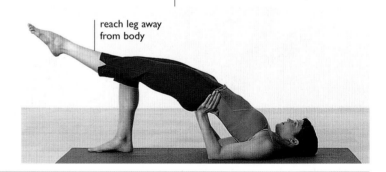

reach leg away from body

At a glance

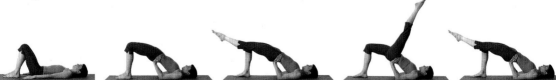

Breathe naturally...Inhale to kick........Exhale to lower..........................Repeat

3 Inhale and toss the leg up high. Exhale and reach it long, lowering it to Step 2 position. As you advance, you may lower the leg further as long as the hips stay level. Repeat 3 times and replace the foot on the mat. Repeat with other leg. TRANSITION: *Release the hands and roll the spine down onto the mat. Use the Preparation exercise* (see pp26–9) *to sit up for the Spine Twist* (see pp 128–129).

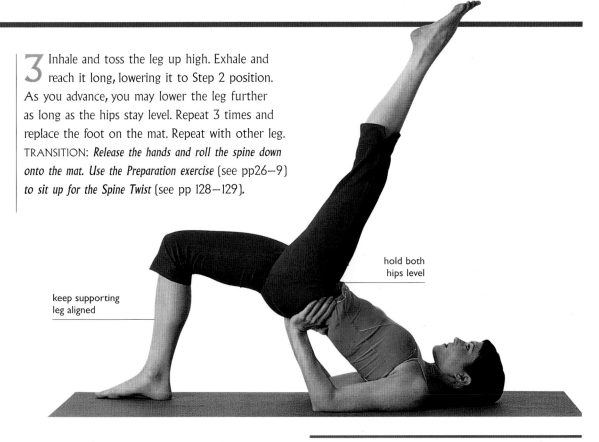

keep supporting leg aligned

hold both hips level

HEAD-TO-TOE CHECKLIST

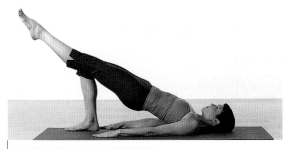

MODIFIED ARM POSITION

If you have difficulty bearing weight on your elbows or wrists, place both arms flat on the mat. Without the hand support, you will need to work harder to maintain the placement of the hips. Hold your box strong, from shoulder to shoulder and from hip to hip.

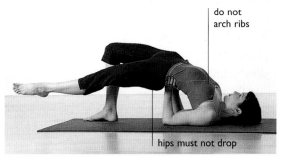

do not arch ribs

hips must not drop

• **Use opposition** – as the leg reaches down, the hips press higher.

• **Kick** swiftly but not forcefully. The motion shouldn't affect your box.

• **Stretch** the leg away from the body as it lowers.

• **Arrange** the hips, knees, and feet in a straight line.

• **As you lift** your hips, your body weight shifts slightly to the shoulders.

• **Lower** the leg to the body's midline. Don't let it drift from the centre line.

SPINE TWIST

The Spine Twist brings you right side up again after a series of inverted exercises. Work your waistline, focusing on lifting up and lengthening the area between your hipbones and your rib cage. The muscles of your spine will stretch as well as those at the backs of the legs. Finally, remember to breathe.

REPETITIONS Repeat entire sequence 3–5 times.

CAUTION Omit this exercise if you have a recent back injury. If you have a bad shoulder, reach back only within a pain-free range.

VISUALIZATION Envision the muscles of your back twisting up around your spine, just like the coloured stripes of an old-fashioned barber's pole.

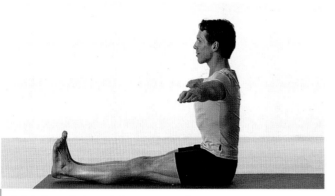

1 Inhale and sit straight up, extending your arms out to the sides, palms down. The legs are straight and held tightly together. All ten toes point up to the ceiling.

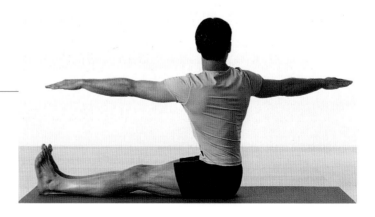

2 Exhale and pivot to one side, twisting your waist with a light double pulse. Look towards your back arm as you turn. As you twist, keep pressing through your heel bones, lifting taller and straighter.

At a glance

 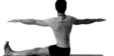 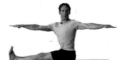

Inhale to sit tall..Exhale to twist...................Rest

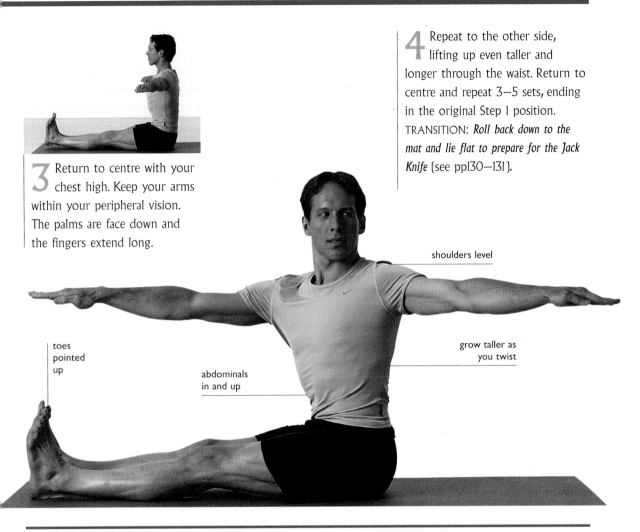

3 Return to centre with your chest high. Keep your arms within your peripheral vision. The palms are face down and the fingers extend long.

4 Repeat to the other side, lifting up even taller and longer through the waist. Return to centre and repeat 3–5 sets, ending in the original Step 1 position.
TRANSITION: *Roll back down to the mat and lie flat to prepare for the Jack Knife* (see pp130–131).

shoulders level

toes pointed up

abdominals in and up

grow taller as you twist

HEAD-TO-TOE CHECKLIST

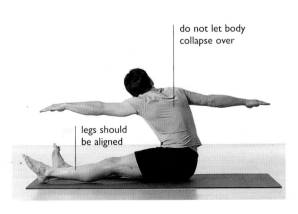

do not let body collapse over

legs should be aligned

• **Do not** allow the back shoulder to hunch up when turning.

• **The arms** remain within your peripheral vision. Do not swing the arms wildly, especially when twisting.

• **Anchor** your sit-bones into the mat. You must not adjust one hip forwards as you turn your waist – all the work happens above the waist.

• **Align** your heel bones and keep them together. If one foot slides forwards, it means you have changed your hip position.

• **Exhale** completely. Wring out all the air from the lungs each time you twist around.

JACK KNIFE

By now you should be comfortable with lifting your hips overhead. The Jack Knife is designed to shift your focus from lifting up to lowering down. A controlled descent from an overhead position is a true indicator of Pilates strength. Control your centre and you will control the exercise.

> **REPETITIONS** 3 times.
>
> **CAUTION** Do not perform this exercise if you have a delicate neck. Certain shoulder injuries may be aggravated by this exercise.
>
> **VISUALIZATION** As you begin your descent, imagine someone cupping your heels and firmly pushing you down. Gently resist as you roll through the spine.

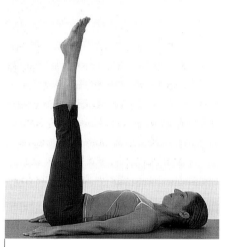

1 Lie on your back with the arms long and both legs straight up to the ceiling. The shoulders and palms press firmly down into the mat. Relax the ribs and scoop the navel towards the spine.

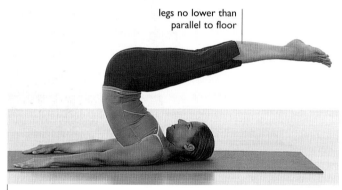

legs no lower than parallel to floor

2 Inhale and use the powerhouse to lift the hips off the mat, carrying the legs overhead into a shallow "pike" position. Continue to lengthen the neck and do not allow the shoulders to curl up off the mat.

At a glance

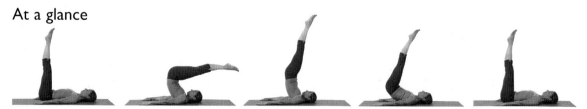

Breathe naturally.........................Inhale.............Exhale...................Repeat

3 Lift your hips even higher, pressing up into a shoulder stand. Extend both legs upwards towards the ceiling, using the strength of your buttocks to support your position. At the peak of the exercise, your feet should be directly over your eyes as the legs rotate together tightly in Pilates stance. The arms continue to press firmly into the mat.

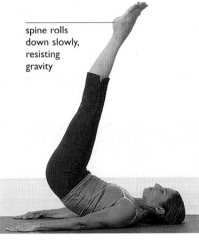

spine rolls
down slowly,
resisting
gravity

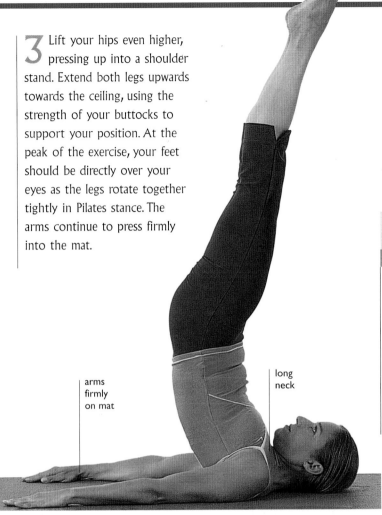

arms
firmly
on mat

long
neck

4 Exhale and angle the legs slightly lower. Begin to roll down through the spine, resisting the descent. Do not allow the feet to fall behind the head as you lower. Finish with both legs at 90° (as in Step 1) and repeat. TRANSITION: *Bend both knees in and roll to one side for the Intermediate Side Kick Series* (see pp98–105).

HEAD-TO-TOE CHECKLIST

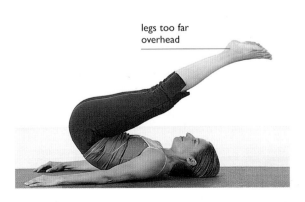

legs too far
overhead

• **Anchor** the back of the head, shoulders, and palms solidly into the mat.
• **Distribute** your weight between the shoulders – not on the neck.
• **During Step 2,** aim the toes for the wall behind you. The legs go no lower than parallel to the floor.
• **Be energetic.** The legs

should press up snappily.
• **On the** descent, keep the feet over the eyes.
• **As the buttocks** reach the mat, the legs remain at a 90° angle to the body. Do not lower them towards the floor or try to swing them over the head as you roll down.

SIDE KICKS: DOUBLE LEG LIFT

This is an exercise in isolation and balance. Your job is to avoid recruiting other muscle groups and, instead, work only the powerhouse. Remember that, seen from above, your body is positioned at an angle. Focus on maintaining that angle as you lower and lift the legs.

REPETITIONS 3–5 times (Steps 2 and 3). *Note: The entire Side Kicks Series is performed to one side before switching to the other leg.*

CAUTION If you experience any neck, shoulder, or wrist pain, extend your bottom arm along the mat and rest your head (see p99).

VISUALIZATION Imagine the hook of a huge crane effortlessly raising your legs up.

1 Lie in the Side Kicks position, with your legs at a 45° angle. Place your free hand on the mat in front of you with the forearm held snugly against your waistline.

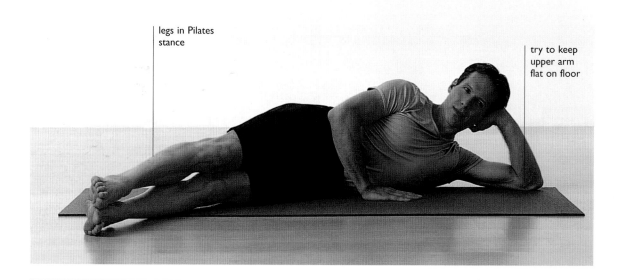

legs in Pilates stance

try to keep upper arm flat on floor

At a glance

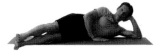 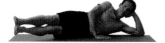 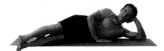

Breathe naturally...Rest

2 In one motion, engage the abdominals and
waistline to float both legs up in the air.
Press the legs together and maintain their angle
in front of the body. Do not rely upon the hand
on the mat. Hold for 3 counts.

neck and
shoulders
relaxed

legs maintain
their angle

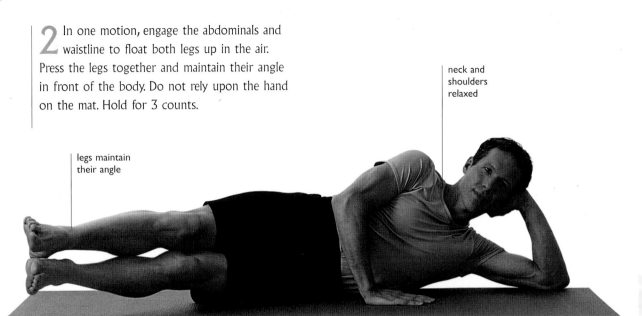

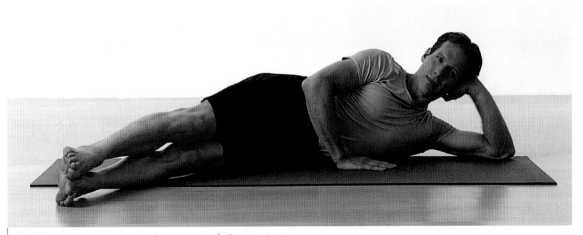

3 Replace your legs on the mat, carefully positioning
them without losing control. Avoid any tendency
to tuck the hips, which will cause them to slide forwards.
Repeat 3–5 times, increasing the height of the legs with
each repetition. Return to Step 1 position to finish.
TRANSITION: *Move on to the Side Kicks: Single Leg Lift*
(see pp134–135).

SIDE KICKS: SINGLE LEG LIFT

Continuing the theme of muscle isolation, the Single Leg Lift targets the inner thighs. Performed in combination with the Double Leg Lift (*see pp132–133*), these movements also improve coordination and train you to move continuously, threading each exercise together. Move precisely without gripping your leg muscles.

REPETITIONS 4–6 times (Steps 2–3). *Note: The entire Side Kicks Series is performed to one side before switching to the other leg.*

CAUTION If you experience any neck, shoulder, or wrist pain, adopt modified position (see p99).

VISUALIZATION Imagine your legs as fireplace bellows. Squeeze them together as though you were pushing out the air in the bellows.

1 Continue directly on from the Double Leg Lift. Lie on your side with your legs extended out at a 45° angle in front of you. The hand of the upper arm is flat on the mat.

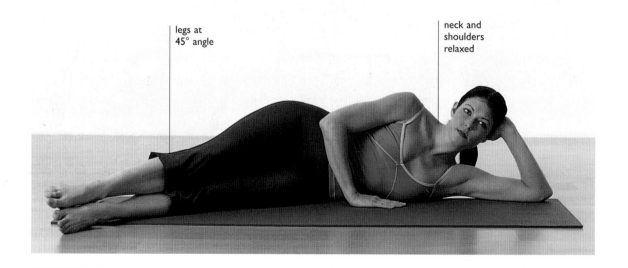

legs at 45° angle

neck and shoulders relaxed

At a glance

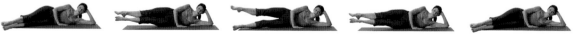

Breathe naturally..Rest

2 Elevate both legs without allowing them
to drift backwards. The angle of the body
should remain constant and the underside of the
supporting arm should stay flush on the mat.
Do not tense the neck or shoulders.

legs remain at
45° angle to body

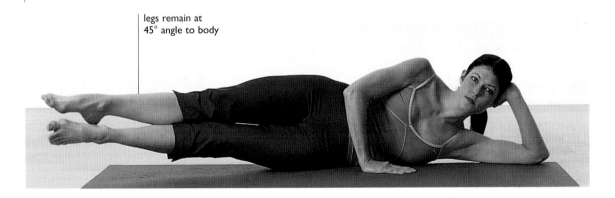

work in Pilates
stance

inner thighs
working

navel pulled
in to spine

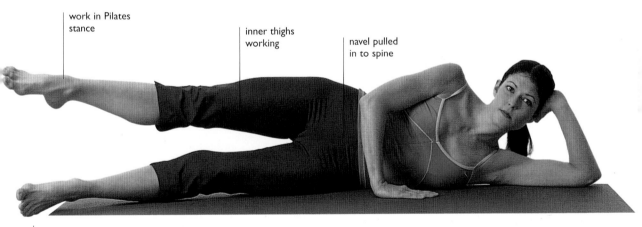

3 Without moving the upper leg, lower the
bottom leg towards the mat. Lift and lower
for 4–6 repetitions, gently squeezing the inner
thighs together each time. Keep wrapping the backs
of the legs together to work the buttocks. Lower
both legs to their starting position to finish.
TRANSITION: *Remain as you are for the Side Kicks:
Bicycle* (see pp136–137).

SIDE KICKS: BICYCLE

This is the last exercise in the Side Kicks Series that we will cover. You should have activated your core muscles in the two preceding exercises and this large movement will challenge that core control. Focus on maintaining your posture and holding your balance in spite of the sweeping motion of the leg.

> **REPETITIONS** Pedal 2–3 times in each direction. *Note: The entire Side Kicks Series is performed to one side before switching to the other leg.*
>
> **CAUTION** If you experience any neck, shoulder, or wrist pain, extend your lower arm along the mat and rest your head (see p99).
>
> **VISUALIZATION** Imagine your leg pedaling a huge bicycle forwards and backwards.

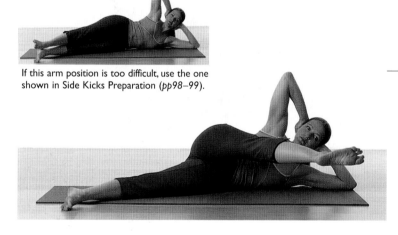

If this arm position is too difficult, use the one shown in Side Kicks Preparation (pp98–99).

1 Lie on your side with your hand behind your head and your elbow pointed towards the ceiling. Carry the top leg forwards as high as possible, keeping it parallel to the floor.

2 At the leg's highest point, bend the knee in tightly towards the shoulder. The heel should aim towards the buttocks. Keep the leg in proper alignment. The hip, knee, and ankle are at the same level. Open the chest and keep your eyes straight ahead.

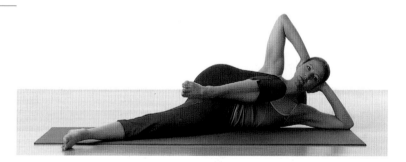

At a glance

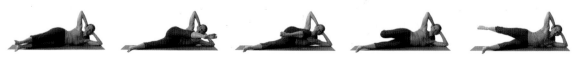

Breathe naturally throughout...Repeat

3 Sweep the knee down in line with the other knee without disrupting or changing your upper body. Now carry the thigh even further back, keeping the foot glued to the buttocks and pressing the hip forwards. The bottom foot remains pressed into the floor.

leg parallel to floor

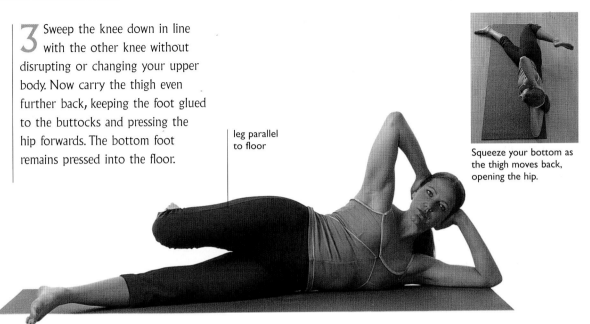

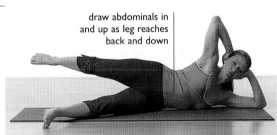

Squeeze your bottom as the thigh moves back, opening the hip.

4 With the upper leg behind you, extend the foot back and down, straightening the leg. Repeat 2–3 times then pedal in the opposite direction 2–3 times. TRANSITION: *Roll onto your stomach for the Transition Heel Beats (see pp138–139) before repeating the Side Kicks Series with the other leg. Then lie on your back for the Intermediate Teaser Series (see pp106–109).*

draw abdominals in and up as leg reaches back and down

HEAD-TO-TOE CHECKLIST

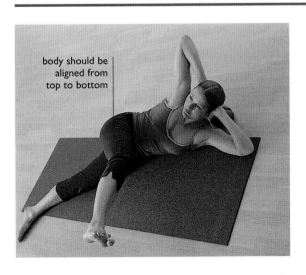

body should be aligned from top to bottom

• **Align** your body from top to bottom. The shoulders and hips remain stacked. Avoid shifting or leaning forwards or back.

• **Hold** your upper arm still to help you control your trunk.

• **During Step 4** press your hip forwards in opposition to the leg stretching back. Tighten the crease where the buttock meets the thigh.

• **Work** the pedaling leg in parallel. To gauge your placement, make sure the leg is working in line with the hip.

• **Modify** the exercise if you have difficulty maintaining your balance. Place the top hand on the mat for added stability.

TRANSITION: HEEL BEATS

This movement is a wonderful example of the efficiency of the Pilates method in using actual exercises to change positions. Use this transitional exercise both here and in the intermediate workout after the Side Kicks: Circles (*see pp 104–105*) to take you smoothly from one side to the other.

REPETITIONS 10–20 beats.

CAUTION If a shoulder or elbow injury causes you pain or discomfort in this position, try turning your palms face up.

VISUALIZATION Suspend your legs above the floor as though you were trying to keep them above water.

1 Begin face down and place your head on your hands. Rotate into Pilates stance by tightening your buttocks and squeezing the backs of the legs together from the inner thighs down to the heels.

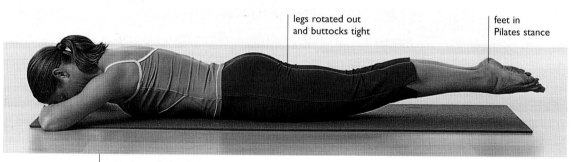

legs rotated out and buttocks tight

feet in Pilates stance

2 Stretch both legs long and straight and lift them just above the mat. Keep the upper body relaxed. Maintain your rotation in Pilates stance while the feet remain long and loose.

At a glance

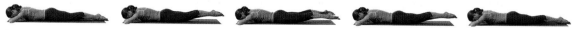

Breathe naturally..Rest

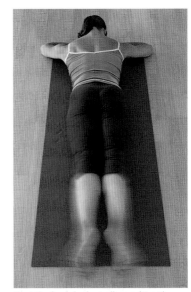

3 Beat the inner thighs and heels vigorously for 10–20 counts. Stretch right through the toes Lower the legs to Step 1 position to finish. TRANSITION: *Roll onto your other side to repeat the entire Side Kicks Series, starting with the Intermediate Series (see pp98–105). When finished, roll onto your back for the Intermediate Teaser Series (see pp140–143).*

Beat the legs rhythmically, working the muscles of the buttocks and inner thighs.

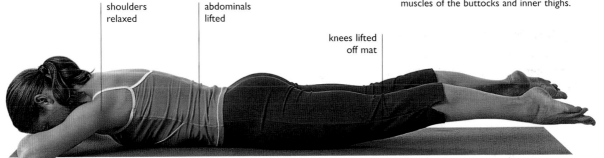

shoulders
relaxed

abdominals
lifted

knees lifted
off mat

HEAD-TO-TOE CHECKLIST

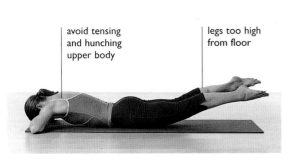

avoid tensing
and hunching
upper body

legs too high
from floor

- **Work** the abdominals to support the lower back. Even in this position, the stomach muscles should be lifted.
- **As you lift** the legs off the mat, don't grip or tense the lower back muscles.
- **The legs** work just above floor level.

- **Synchronize** the legs: they should open and close at the same time and at the same height.
- **Relax** the upper body: avoid hunching or rounding the shoulders.
- **The heels** beat lightly. It is the work of the inner thighs that is the focal point of the exercise.

TEASER 2

This exercise is a variation on a theme. In Teaser 1 (*see pp108–109*), we fix the legs in space and move the body up and down. Now we do just the opposite: the upper body remains still as the legs move up and down. Working at this angle targets the lower part of the abdominals. Begin small and gradually increase.

REPETITIONS 1 set (3–5 lifts).

CAUTION If you have a weak or injured back, omit this exercise or proceed with caution.

VISUALIZATION Imagine your legs mimicking the action of a ball on a trampoline, rebounding up with each lift.

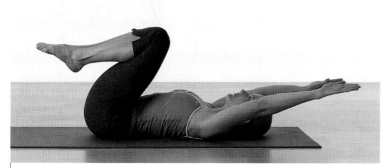

1 Begin on your back with knees drawn in and arms above your ears. Lengthen your spine on the mat and hold your ribs in. You may begin this exercise from the last upright position of Teaser 1. In this case, skip now to Step 3.

2 Extend both legs to 45° without changing your spine. Inhale and initiate as you did the Teaser 1, gradually peeling up off the mat.

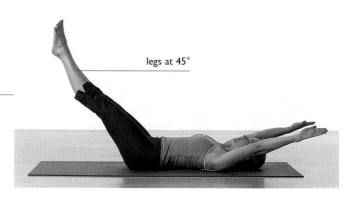

legs at 45°

At a glance

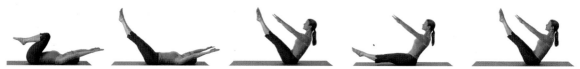

Breathe naturally...............................Inhale to lower legs........Exhale to lift

3 Exhale and sit up in a perfect "V" shape, reaching the fingers for the toes. Find a balance point where you can move the legs independently of the body. Leaning too far forwards or back will compromise your stability. Be certain to keep scooping back in the waistline, and work the legs in Pilates stance.

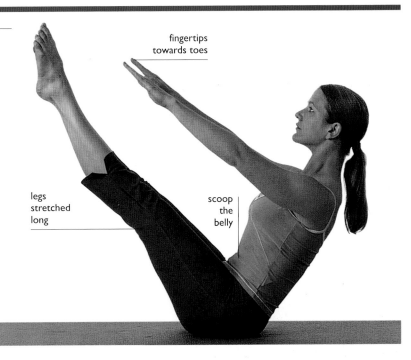

fingertips
towards toes

legs
stretched
long

scoop
the
belly

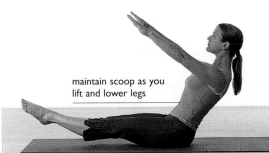

maintain scoop as you
lift and lower legs

4 Without leaning back, lower and lift the legs the legs 3–5 times, exhaling on each lift. Roll down and return to Step 1 position to rest.
TRANSITION: *For an advanced transition on your final leg lift, raise both arms overhead. Roll down to the mat, reaching the arms back and the legs forwards simultaneously to prepare for Teaser 3 (see pp142–143).*

HEAD-TO-TOE CHECKLIST

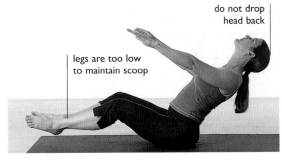

do not drop
head back

legs are too low
to maintain scoop

• **Begin** with small movements. Lowering your legs beyond your point of control can cause you to arch your back and bulge your abdominals.

• **Check** that your head stays in line with your spine. Don't lean back as your legs lower.

• **The arms** work parallel to the legs. Use the reaching action of the arms to counteract any tendency to lean back.

• **If you have** difficulty lowering the legs, you may soften the knees slightly, but keep the toes above the knees at all times (see *p109*).

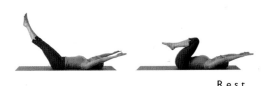

. . . . R e s t

TEASER 3

This is the culmination of the two preceding Teaser exercises and requires enormous control. During Teaser 1, we held the legs steady and worked the upper body; in Teaser 2, we reversed that pattern. Here we simultaneously move the upper and the lower body, developing coordination as well as stamina.

REPETITIONS Repeat entire sequence 3 times.

CAUTION Omit the exercise or proceed with caution if you have a weak or injured back.

VISUALIZATION Imagine your body being pulled apart by your fingers and toes like a rubber band. The moment before you arrive on the mat, you snap together again.

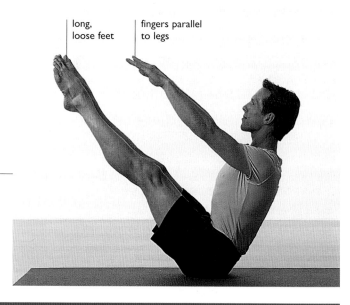

1 Following the end of Teaser 2 (*see pp140–141*), the arms are overhead. Lower the body smoothly down towards the mat, reaching the arms and legs out. Stop when the limbs arrive just above the mat.

long, loose feet

fingers parallel to legs

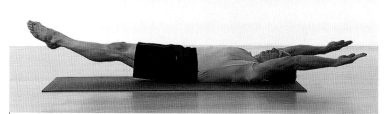

2 As your limbs approach the floor, inhale and swiftly fold your body up into a perfect "V" shape. Balance on your tailbone and reach the fingers to the toes, scooping the abdominals in towards the spine.

At a glance

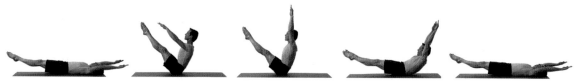

Inhale....................Exhale............Inhale............Exhale........................Repeat

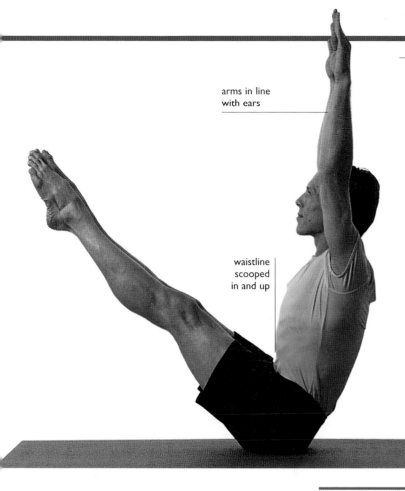

arms in line
with ears

waistline
scooped
in and up

3 Sweep both arms overhead, directly in line with your ears. Do not change the position of the spine or the legs. Lift tall, lengthening the waistline. As you move onto Step 4, make sure that the arms remain behind the ears.

4 Exhale as you simultaneously lower the arms and legs down to the mat. Repeat the sequence twice more. To finish, lower down to the mat and hug the knees or move onto the next exercise.
TRANSITION: *Hold your final Teaser and lower the arms down and back to place the hands on the mat. Keep the legs as high as possible to prepare for the Can–Can (see pp144–145) or Advanced Hip Circles (see pp146–147).*

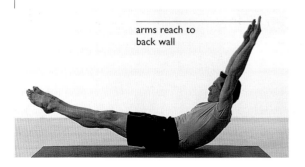

arms reach to
back wall

HEAD-TO-TOE CHECKLIST

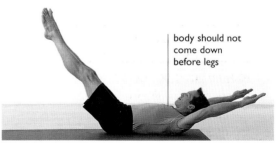

body should not
come down
before legs

• **Do not** allow the upper body to arrive on the mat before the lower body and legs – or vice versa.
• **Vary** the dynamics. Stretch out long and slow; rise up quick and easy.

• **Work** at threshold (see p19) – if you move too quickly, you may sacrifice your powerhouse.
• **Wrap** the backs of the legs together to maintain Pilates stance.

CAN-CAN

This is a preparatory exercise for the Hip Circles (*see pp146–147*). Perform the sequence rhythmically and focus on opening the chest and shoulders. Think of the dancers in a French chorus line and keep in time with their high-kicking legs. The taller you lift up, the easier this exercise will become.

REPETITIONS 2–3 sets of alternating sides.

CAUTION If you have a wrist injury, you may prop back on your elbows. If you feel strain in your hip sockets, place the soles of your feet on the mat and continue.

VISUALIZATION As you kick, envision yourself sitting with your back against a tall tree. Keep upright.

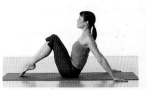

Place your hands behind you and bend your knees in.

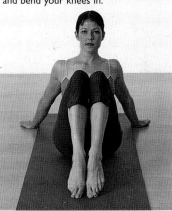

1 Sit up tall, with your knees drawn in to your chest. The tiptoes rest on the mat. Place your hands behind you, a little wider than the shoulders.

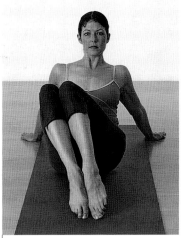

2 Keeping the waist lifted, twist the legs to the right. The knees will roll to the side, angling down towards the ground. Hands are pressed firmly into the floor behind you. Do not let the lower back sink down or tuck under.

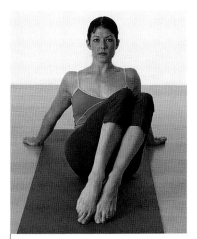

3 Now twist to the left, continuing to lift tall in the upper body. Keep your position tight and close, with the knees folded in towards the body and tiptoes light on the mat.

At a glance

Breathe naturally..............................Exhale to kick up....Repeat

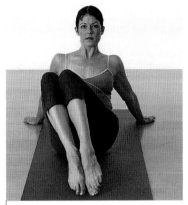

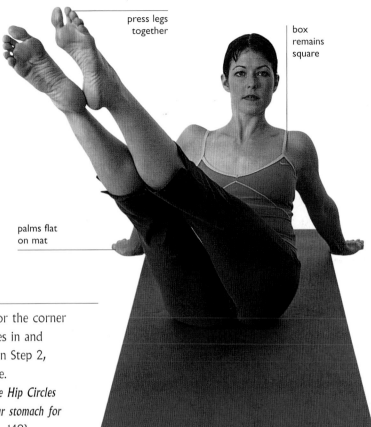

press legs together

box remains square

palms flat on mat

4 Twist to the right one last time. To ensure that the legs do not drift further from your body with each twist, keep the heels close to the buttocks.

5 Kick both legs up, aiming for the corner behind you. Bend both knees in and replace the toes on the mat, as in Step 2, ready to repeat to the other side.
TRANSITION: *Move directly into the Hip Circles* (see pp 146–147) *or turn onto your stomach for the Advanced Swimming* (see pp148–149).

HEAD-TO-TOE CHECKLIST

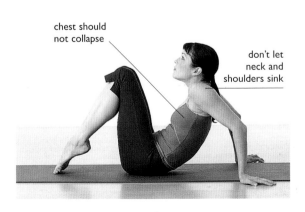

chest should not collapse

don't let neck and shoulders sink

• **Don't collapse** in your neck or shoulders. Aim the crown of the head towards the ceiling.
• **Keep lengthening** your waist. Think of increasing the distance between the top of your hips and the bottom of your ribs.
• **Your arms** are straight, but not locked, in order to protect the wrists.

• **As you** twist your knees, do not turn your upper body.
• **Aim as** high as possible, ideally taking your legs up towards one ear.
• **Press** the knees together as you "can-can" from side to side.

HIP CIRCLES

Often referred to as Teaser 4, the Hip Circles is one of the most challenging exercises in the advanced routine. The abdominal wall stabilizes your torso as you sweep your legs in a circle, all the while balancing on your tailbone. Though presented as step-by-step instructions, the exercise moves continuously without pauses.

REPETITIONS 2–3 sets, alternating direction of circles.

CAUTION Perform this exercise cautiously if you have a delicate back or have suffered a recent back injury. If you have a weak shoulder, lower onto your elbows.

VISUALIZATION Imagine that you are a gymnast working on the parallel bars. The legs sweep around as the arms support the body.

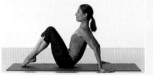
Hands are wider than shoulders and fingers point away from body.

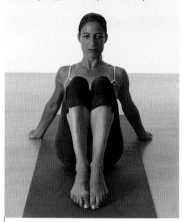

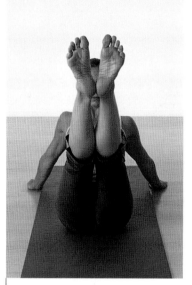

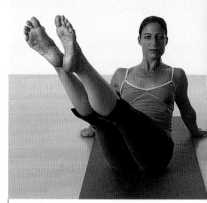

1 Begin as you did the Can-Can (*see pp144–145*) with the knees bent and tiptoes on the mat. From the end of Teaser 3 (*see pp142–143*), skip directly to Step 2 to begin.

2 Stretch both legs up directly in front of you into a Teaser position. To avoid sinking backwards, keep your back tall and your chest lifted. The legs should lift as high as possible, folding the body in half.

3 Fasten your legs together and inhale as you circle them to the right side. Hold the upper body still by drawing the waistline in and up, activating your "girdle of strength".

At a glance

Inhale to circle down........Exhale to circle up.........Repeat in reverse direction

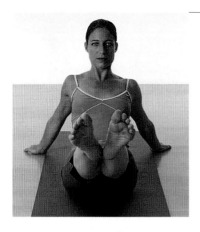

4 Carry the legs down and around through the centre line. Keep the legs within your control. If your back arches or your waistline distends, your legs have gone too low. Work within a smaller range until your strength increases.

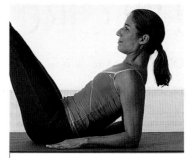

MODIFIED ARM POSITION

If you have an injured shoulder or wrist, you may perform this exercise supported on your elbows rather than your hands.

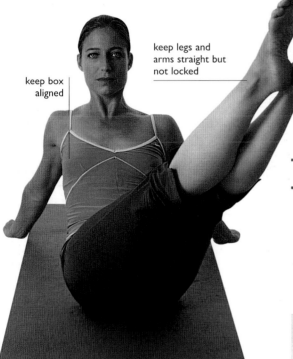

keep box aligned

keep legs and arms straight but not locked

HEAD-TO-TOE CHECKLIST

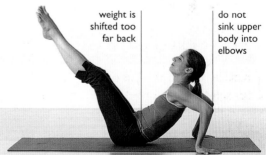

weight is shifted too far back

do not sink upper body into elbows

5 Exhale and circle the legs up to the left. Return them to centre, aiming first behind the left ear and then to the midline. Repeat 2–3 times, alternating the direction of each circle. Focus on lifting the legs progressively higher with each repetition.

TRANSITION: *Bend both knees in and turn onto your stomach to prepare for the Swimming* (see pp148–149).

- **Begin** small, increasing the circles as you gain strength.
- **Circle** only as large as can be controlled – taking the legs too low will compromise your scoop.
- **Do not** let the upper body collapse. Keep the chest open and neck long.
- **Press** the wings down and back to avoid sinking backwards.
- **Circle** dynamically, accenting the upswing of the circle.

SWIMMING

The intense abdominal work of the Teasers makes it necessary to address the flip side of the body again. This exercise lengthens the stomach muscles while strengthening the back muscles. As you near the end of the matwork, remember the more basic principles of powerhouse support and working within your frame.

REPETITIONS 10–20 counts.

CAUTION A shoulder injury may be aggravated by this exercise. Reduce the range of motion of the arms, or omit the exercise. Those with lower back injuries should approach this exercise carefully.

VISUALIZATION Envision your legs working as if using a float in a swimming pool.

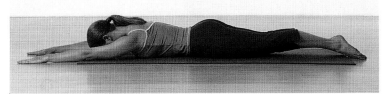

1 Lie face down, outstretched on the mat. Even in this position you should be actively lifting your abdominals. Squeeze the backs of the legs together and reach the arms long on the mat.

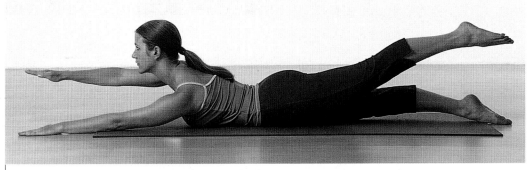

2 Lift your head and then your right arm and left leg. The thigh muscles tighten to stretch the legs. Stretch out long and thin, lengthening your lower back. Breathe naturally throughout.

At a glance

Breathe naturally throughout...Rest

3 Without shifting your body weight, flutter the arms and legs in a swimming motion for 10–20 counts. Return to Step 1 position to finish. To stretch your lower back, sit back on your heels in child's pose (*see p93*).
TRANSITION: *Roll up to kneeling and assume a push-up position for the Leg Pull Down* (see pp150–151).

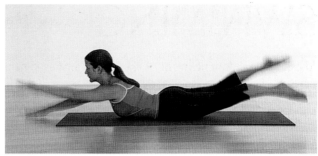

Move rapidly and keep your head up as though you were actually in water.

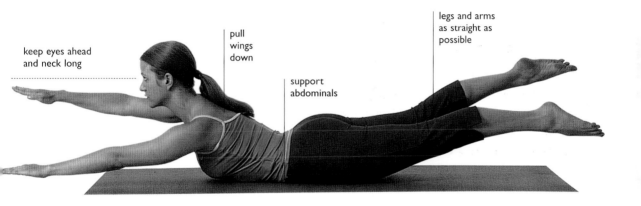

keep eyes ahead and neck long

pull wings down

support abdominals

legs and arms as straight as possible

HEAD-TO-TOE CHECKLIST

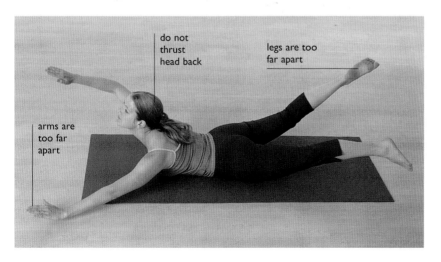

do not thrust head back

legs are too far apart

arms are too far apart

• **Hold** your gaze high without crunching the back of your neck.
• **Work** the arms directly in front of you and in line with your shoulders.
• **The legs** should flutter close to each other and in line with your torso.
• **Swim** briskly but avoid rocking from side to side.

LEG PULL DOWN

This exercise is one of the most advanced Pilates movements. In a push-up position you reduce the surfaces upon which you bear weight to only the hands and feet. Thus the powerhouse becomes entirely responsible for all the work you do. Hold strong in your centre, moving your body in one rigid piece.

REPETITIONS 2–3 sets of alternating legs.

CAUTION Omit this exercise if you are unable to bear weight on your hands or wrists. Modify the movement for an ankle injury by keeping both feet on the mat and stretching the heels back and forth.

VISUALIZATION Imagine pressing your body back, aiming your supporting heel to the floor.

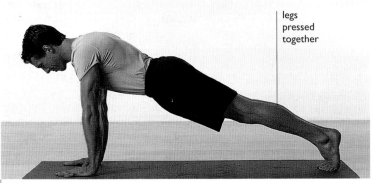

legs pressed together

1 Establish a push-up position with your legs pressed tightly together and your abdominals lifted. From head to heels your body should resemble a plank.

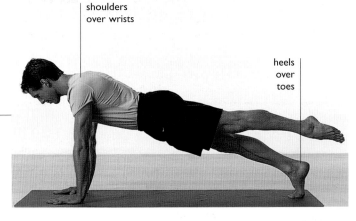

shoulders over wrists

heels over toes

2 Inhale and raise one leg behind you, reaching it towards the back of the room. Don't shift your body weight to one side but keep centred and lift the abdominals.

At a glance

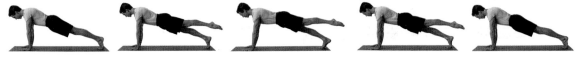

Breathe naturally...Inhale..........Exhale.............Inhale......Repeat to other side

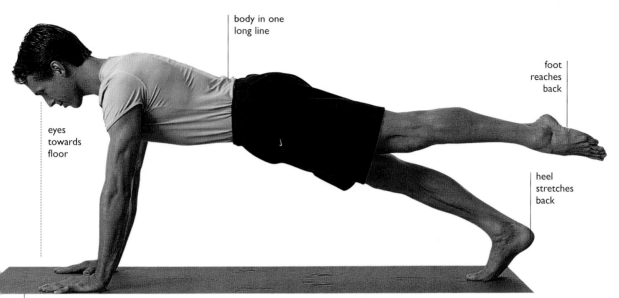

body in one
long line

foot
reaches
back

eyes
towards
floor

heel
stretches
back

3 Exhale and stretch the standing heel back for two pulses. Lift the heel back up and replace the outstretched leg before repeating with the other leg. TRANSITION: *Flip onto your back and sit up tall for the Leg Pull Up (see pp152–153). For an advanced transition to this exercise, walk one* hand into the centre of the mat and release the other hand, extending it sideways and back. Pivot your body up to the ceiling until you can replace your hand on the mat underneath you. The hips remain in the air (see p152, Step 2). The feet adjust on the mat so that the heels are down and the fingers must point to the toes.

HEAD-TO-TOE CHECKLIST

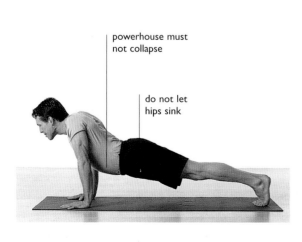

powerhouse must
not collapse

do not let
hips sink

• **Lift** your centre. The hips must not drop at any point.
• **Do not sink** into your shoulders. Focus on keeping a broad, flat upper back.
• **Stretch** each leg back with a smooth but vigorous pulse.
• **Continue** to press the back of the legs together, tightening the buttocks.
• **Plant** your hands firmly on the mat but do not lock or jam the elbows.
• **Your neck** maintains perfect alignment with the rest of the body. Keep the back of the neck long and the head tilted slightly down to avoid jutting the chin forwards.

LEG PULL UP

Remember this exercise as the Leg Pull *facing up*, so as to avoid confusion with the Leg Pull Down (*see pp150–151*). Supported by only your hands and feet, the buttocks and midsection work double duty in this exercise. Move swiftly through the exercise as most of your body weight is on the wrists.

REPETITIONS 2–4 sets (each set comprises 3 kicks with each leg).

CAUTION Omit this exercise if you have an acute shoulder or wrist injury. If your wrists become sore, rest between sets. For an ankle injury, proceed with caution.

VISUALIZATION Imagine your body supported on an inclined ramp. As you toss the leg up, the torso remains supported.

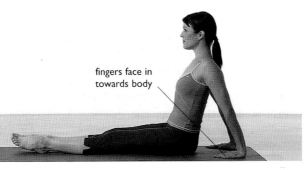

fingers face in towards body

1 Sit upright with the legs long and straight and your hands on the mat behind you. Draw the backs of the legs together to begin.

2 Press your hips up, establishing a reverse push-up position. Look straight ahead and tighten your buttocks, positioning yourself in one long line.

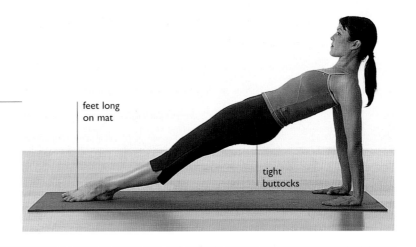

feet long on mat

tight buttocks

At a glance

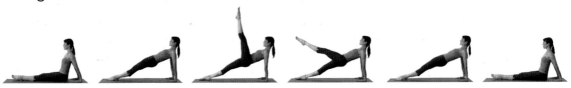

Inhale...................................Exhale............................Inhale..............Rest

3 Toss one leg up as high as possible. Keep your hips lifted so that your entire body is level. The leg aims straight up towards the midline of the body. As you kick up, be certain your supporting leg does not roll outwards towards the ankle bone.

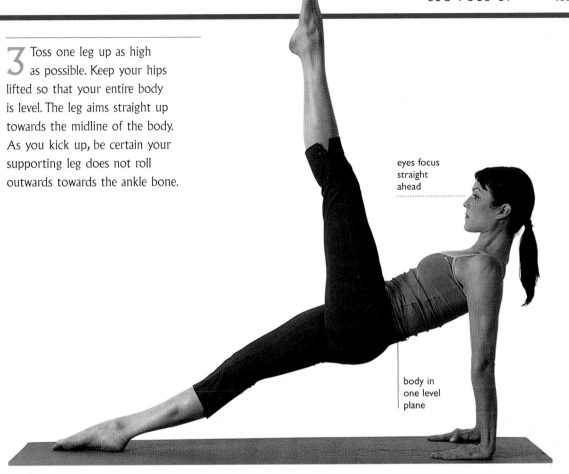

eyes focus straight ahead

body in one level plane

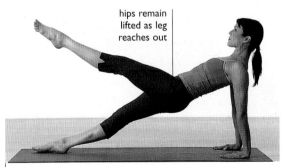

hips remain lifted as leg reaches out

4 Lower the leg, without sinking the pelvis, and kick it up twice more. Switch legs; repeat 2–4 sets. Lower hips and return to Step 1 position to rest. TRANSITION: *With your hips still raised, bend one knee and slide it under you. Transfer your weight onto your knees, pivoting to face one side of your mat for the Kneeling Side Kicks (see pp154–155).*

HEAD-TO-TOE CHECKLIST

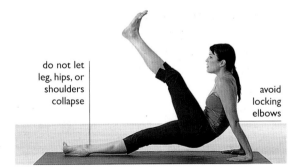

do not let leg, hips, or shoulders collapse

avoid locking elbows

- **Press** your shoulders down and lengthen your neck.
- **Keep** your limbs straight, but not locked.

- **Use** your girdle of strength to keep your hips lifted.
- **Heels** remain on the mat even if the toes do not.

KNEELING SIDE KICKS

This exercise will challenge your balance and tone your waistline. Similar to the Side Kicks: Front (*see pp100–101*), the Kneeling Side Kicks is impossible to perform without proper alignment. Imagine seeing yourself from the ceiling, in one long line from head to toe. Begin with small controlled movements.

REPETITIONS 3 times with each leg.

CAUTION Eliminate this exercise if you are unable to kneel or if you have an acute wrist injury.

VISUALIZATION In your initial position (Step 2), try to envision your entire body sandwiched between two walls.

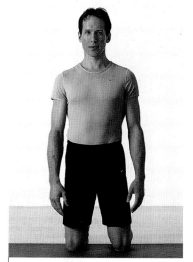

2 Place your left hand on the mat directly underneath the shoulder and the right hand behind the head. Lift the right leg up, stretching it long.

1 From the end of the Leg Pull Up (*see pp152–153*), shift into an upright, kneeling position. You should be centred on your mat, facing its long edge.

The elevated leg is in line with the body.

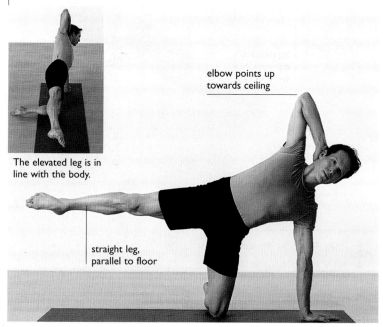

elbow points up towards ceiling

straight leg, parallel to floor

At a glance

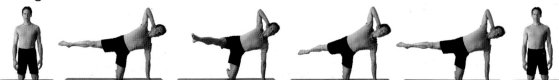

Breathe naturally....Inhale to kick forward........Exhale to kick back..........Rest

3 Carry the leg forwards, parallel to the ground. As it reaches its highest point, kick it twice with a double pulse. As you kick, maintain your shoulder over your hand and your hip over your knee. Do not allow the ribs to protrude or the foot on the mat to adjust its position.

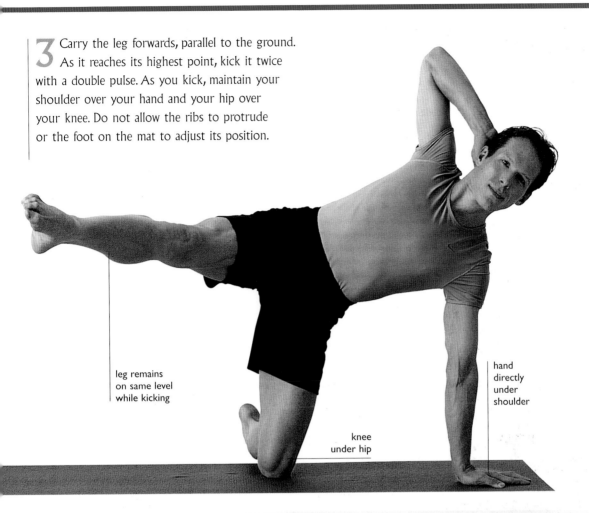

leg remains on same level while kicking

hand directly under shoulder

knee under hip

4 Now take the leg behind you without distending the belly or ribs. Work the opposition — as the leg reaches back, the hips press forwards. Kick front and back twice more. Kneel upright as in Step 1 then repeat 3 times on the other side. Return to Step 1 position to finish.

TRANSITION: *Lower your hips to the mat, sitting to one side of the knees for the Mermaid* (see pp156–157).

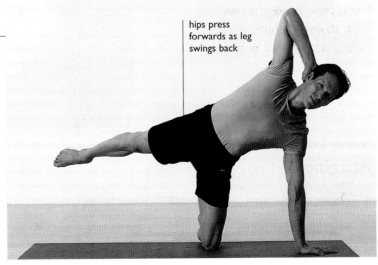

hips press forwards as leg swings back

MERMAID

Designed to stretch the side of the body and create space between the ribs, the Mermaid is an exercise in opposition. Anchor your lower body to the mat and pull your upper body away from it as you reach over your legs. This exercise is a wonderful stretch after working the waist in the Kneeling Side Kicks (*see pp154–155*).

REPETITIONS 2–3 times to each side.

CAUTION Proceed with care if you have an injured knee, hip, or wrist.

VISUALIZATION Imagine yourself reaching for the brass ring in the centre of a merry-go-round. Stretch far away but stay on the horse.

1 Sit tall to one side of your knees. Hug the ankles with one hand and reach the other arm up against the ear.

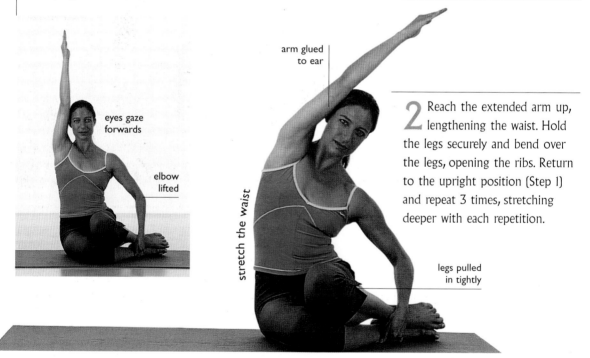

eyes gaze forwards

elbow lifted

arm glued to ear

stretch the waist

2 Reach the extended arm up, lengthening the waist. Hold the legs securely and bend over the legs, opening the ribs. Return to the upright position (Step 1) and repeat 3 times, stretching deeper with each repetition.

legs pulled in tightly

At a glance

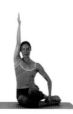
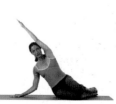
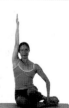

Inhale up......Exhale over......Inhale up.........Exhale over..........Repeat

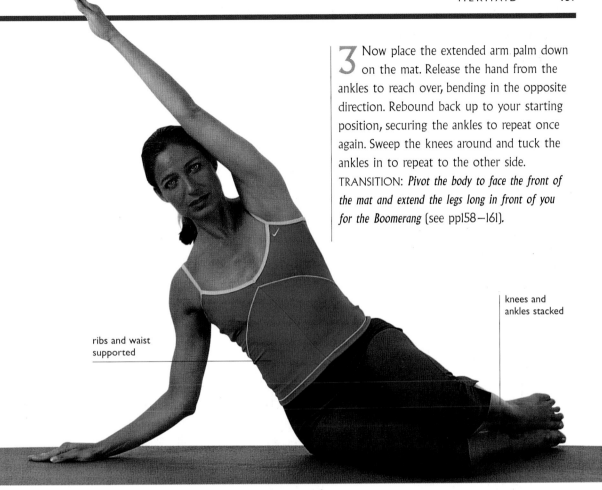

3 Now place the extended arm palm down on the mat. Release the hand from the ankles to reach over, bending in the opposite direction. Rebound back up to your starting position, securing the ankles to repeat once again. Sweep the knees around and tuck the ankles in to repeat to the other side.
TRANSITION: *Pivot the body to face the front of the mat and extend the legs long in front of you for the Boomerang* (see pp158–161).

knees and
ankles stacked

ribs and waist
supported

HEAD-TO-TOE CHECKLIST

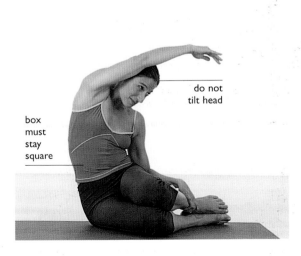

box
must
stay
square

do not
tilt head

• **Keep** square. Focus on your box to properly stretch the muscles of the ribs and waist.
• **Gaze** straight out to keep your head in line with your body.
• **Stretch up** before you stretch over.
• **As you bend** in Step 2, glue the upper arm to the ear – this is the key to the stretch.

• **In Step 3**, your arm on the mat bends very little at first but may increase as you improve.
• **As you** bend away from the feet, keep your ribs and waist lifted.
• **After Step 3,** use your powerhouse to return to your starting position.
• **Stack** the legs. The knees and ankles lie above each other.

BOOMERANG

The Boomerang demonstrates clearly the six classic Pilates principles (*see pp12–13*) in a singular exercise. It is by far the longest piece of choreography in the matwork, combining elements of several different advanced level exercises. This exercise should be one of the very last additions to your routine.

REPETITIONS 4 times.

CAUTION Omit this exercise if you have a history of neck or shoulder injuries.

VISUALIZATION Visualize your body as an object inside a snow globe. Drift slowly and smoothly back and forth without any sudden movements.

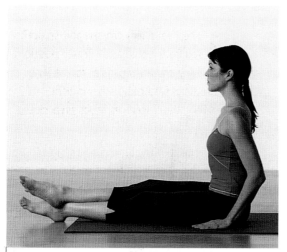

1 Sit in the centre of the mat so that you have enough room to roll back and forth. Sit upright, with both legs extended along the mat. Cross one leg over the other. Place the hands palms down alongside the hips. Draw the abdominals in and up.

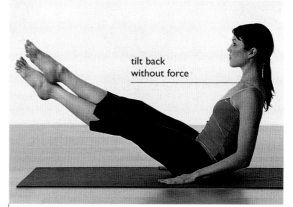

tilt back
without force

2 Initiate from the powerhouse and tip back, bringing the legs instantly off the floor. Inhale and scoop the navel in deeper as you roll back. Do not use your arms to propel yourself backwards.

At a glance

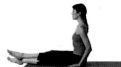 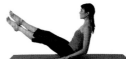 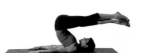 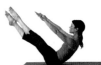

Inhale to begin.......Exhale to roll back........Inhale to switch..................Exhale

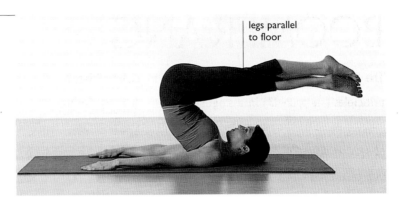

legs parallel
to floor

3 Continue rolling back until your legs are parallel to the floor. Do not roll onto your neck. Exhale as you arrive, pressing the arms firmly into the mat. Swiftly open and close the legs, switching ankles without allowing your hips to sink. In this inverted position there should still be space between your chin and your chest.

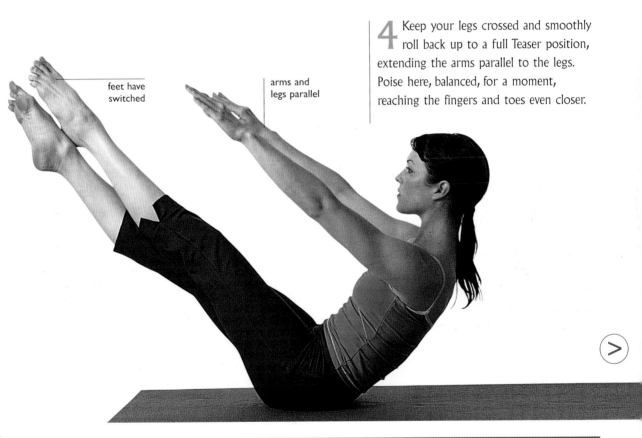

feet have
switched

arms and
legs parallel

4 Keep your legs crossed and smoothly roll back up to a full Teaser position, extending the arms parallel to the legs. Poise here, balanced, for a moment, reaching the fingers and toes even closer.

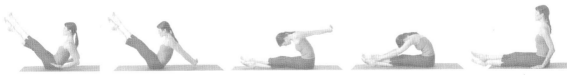

Inhale to stretch arms back.............Exhale to float down.....................Repeat

5 In one motion, turn your palms upwards and bend your elbows into your sides. Continue to reach the legs up and pull your belly button in to your backbone to sustain your position. Elongate the waist to avoid any tendency to tip back as you move into the next step.

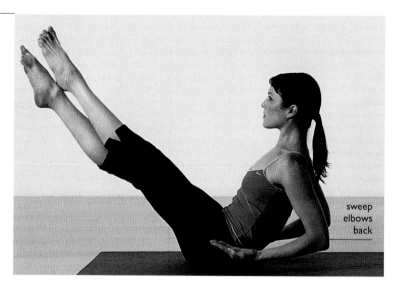

sweep
elbows
back

6 Now bring your arms behind you and secure your hands behind your back, cupping one hand inside the other. Allow the head to lower, tilting the chin downwards. Use your arms as a counterweight, stretching them gently down and back to pull the legs up even higher.

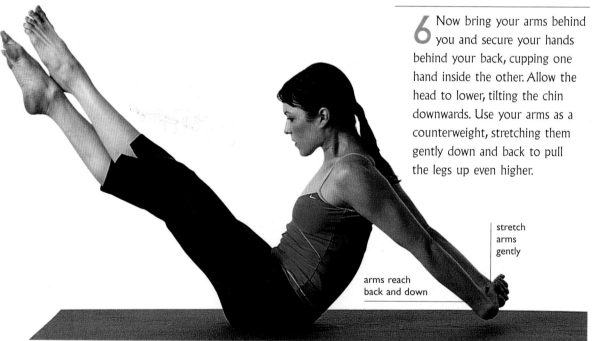

stretch
arms
gently

arms reach
back and down

At a glance

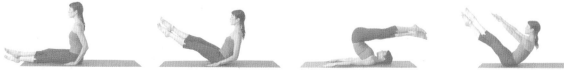

Inhale to begin.......Exhale to roll back........Inhale to switch..................Exhale

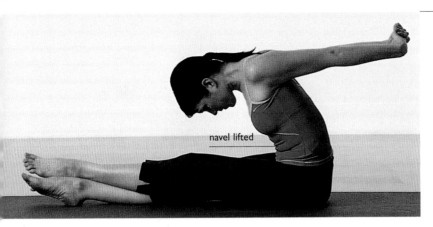

navel lifted

7 Hold this position and float the entire body down onto the mat in front of you. Control your descent, resisting the pull of gravity. As you arrive on the mat, lift your arms up behind you. Keep pulling in the navel.

8 Release the hands and sweep the arms all the way around to rest on the ankles. Roll up to your starting position, placing the hands flat on the mat to begin again. TRANSITION: *Move to the front of the mat to position yourself for the Intermediate Seal* (see pp110–111).

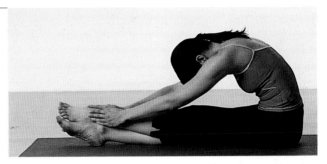

HEAD-TO-TOE CHECKLIST

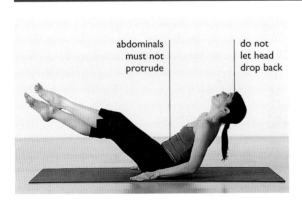

abdominals must not protrude

do not let head drop back

• **Move** continuously – this is one exercise from start to finish.
• **At Step 2**, do not push back forcefully to lift the legs. Activate your power-house to do the work.
• **The body** and legs fold up closer together as you hold your Teaser position.

• **In Step 6**, stretch the arms gently. This is an extreme position and should not be performed quickly or carelessly.
• **Pull** the legs up higher towards the body as you clasp the hands behind the back.

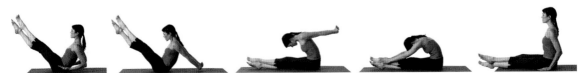

Inhale to stretch arms back.............Exhale to float down.....................Repeat

PUSH UPS

Pilates push ups reinforce the notion that each exercise is designed to work every part of the body. By adjusting the arm position and focusing on the alignment of the spine and neck, you will achieve better results with fewer repetitions than with traditional push ups. This is the last exercise of the Pilates matwork.

REPETITIONS Work up to 3 sets of 3 push ups.

CAUTION Push ups should not be attempted if you have a shoulder, elbow, or wrist injury.

VISUALIZATION In your push up position, envision your body smoothly compressing downwards and briskly rebounding back up.

1 With your legs and feet together in parallel, walk the hands down the body towards the floor. Do not shift your weight back onto your heels.

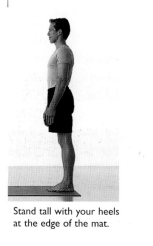

Stand tall with your heels at the edge of the mat.

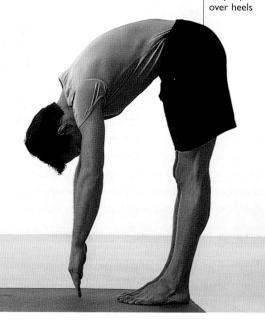

keep hips over heels

At a glance

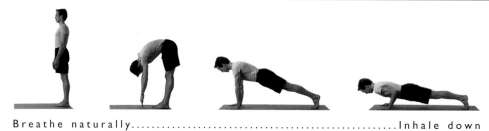

Breathe naturally..Inhale down

2 When your fingers reach the floor, walk the hands out along the mat. Keep your knees as straight as possible and bring your body out into a "push up" position. Your heels are over your toes and shoulders are over your wrists. Lift the abdominals high.

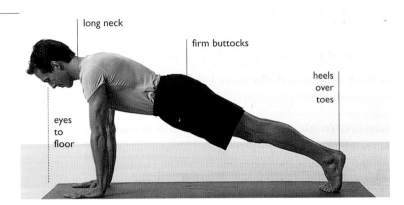

long neck

firm buttocks

heels over toes

eyes to floor

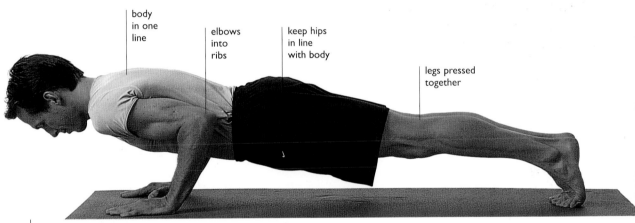

body in one line

elbows into ribs

keep hips in line with body

legs pressed together

3 Perform 3 push ups with the elbows into the sides of the body. To come out of the push up position, lift the powerhouse and fold up in half, pressing the heels into the mat, and walk the hands back to hold the ankles. Give yourself a gentle stretch, pulling the head in towards the shins. Roll up to standing and repeat 2 more sets. On the final repetition, walk the hands back up the body and reach the arms overhead.

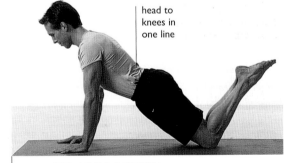

head to knees in one line

MODIFIED LEG POSITION

If you find that you cannot avoid sinking or arching the lower back, bend both knees and kneel on the mat. Or simply begin in the standard position and reduce the range of motion, bending your arms only to your point of control. As you progress, reintroduce the traditional version.

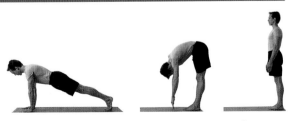

Exhale up...............................Repeat

MAGIC CIRCLE

The Magic Circle is the one truly portable piece of Pilates equipment. A compact, lightweight resistance tool, it is used to target muscles in the arms, legs, and chest as well as those of the powerhouse. As a substitute for a Circle, use a ball 30–40cm (12–16 in) in diameter.

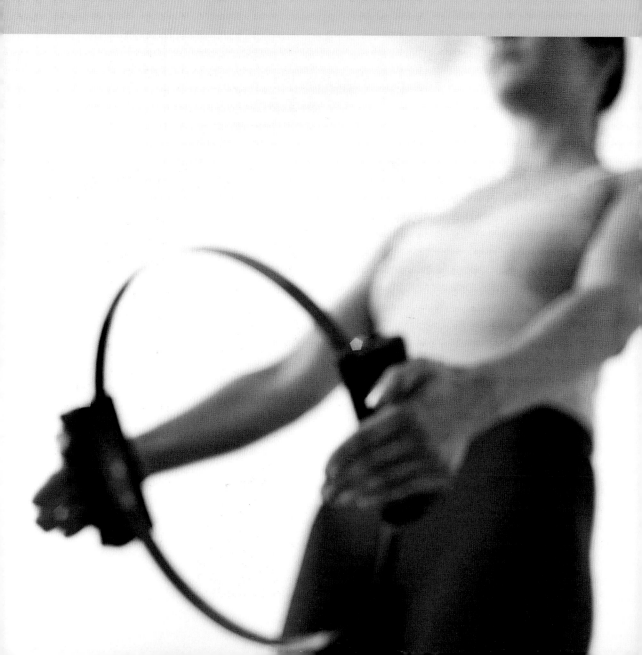

MAGIC CIRCLE: CHEST LEVEL

The Magic Circle exercises demonstrate the classic Pilates blend of lengthening and strengthening. As you perform this exercise, use your centre as the impetus to compress the Circle. Each time you squeeze the Circle, activate your powerhouse and simultaneously focus on lengthening the arms away from you.

Hold the Circle at chest level, with outstretched arms and long fingers. Exhale to compress the Circle. Hold for 3 counts and slowly release with control. Repeat 3–5 times.

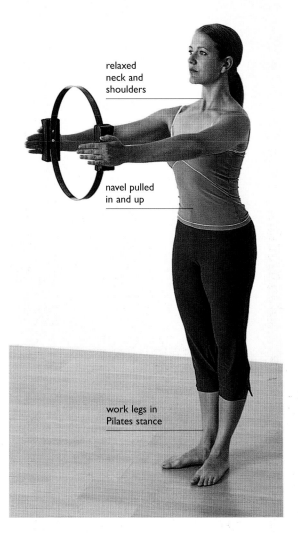

relaxed neck and shoulders

navel pulled in and up

work legs in Pilates stance

HEAD-TO-TOE CHECKLIST

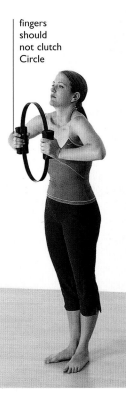

fingers should not clutch Circle

- **Do not** tense the neck and shoulders as you compress the Circle.
- **Avoid** locking the elbows. The arms should be long but loose, and not too close to the body.
- **Cup** the pads of the Circle in the heel of each hand. Fingers remain long – they should not clutch the Circle.
- **Stand** tall and straight. Do not sink back into your heels.
- **The Circle** remains at a fixed distance as you squeeze it.

MAGIC CIRCLE: OVERHEAD

This exercise challenges your ability to sustain your posture and alignment. Shift your weight slightly forwards to lengthen the lower back and continue to lift the waist. Remember, Pilates works your muscles in a lengthened position.

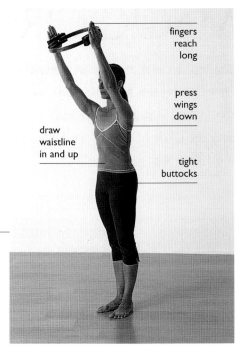

fingers reach long

press wings down

draw waistline in and up

tight buttocks

Establish the Circle over your head within your peripheral vision – if you raise your eyes without tilting your head back you should just be able to see it. Breathe out to compress the Circle for 3 counts and slowly release. Repeat the exercise 3–5 times.

MAGIC CIRCLE: HIP LEVEL

Positioning the Circle lower targets the chest muscles. Imagine it as a basketball hoop; keep it angled enough to allow the ball to swish through the hoop. Focus on pressing the wings down and lengthening the back of the neck.

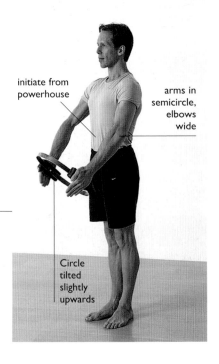

initiate from powerhouse

arms in semicircle, elbows wide

Circle tilted slightly upwards

Position the Circle just below your navel, tilted slightly upwards towards your body. Stretch the fingers long and lift the elbows. Exhale as you squeeze the Circle, keeping it a fixed distance away from the body. Hold it for 3 counts and then release. Repeat 3–5 times, lifting the abdominals and firming the buttocks each time.

MAGIC CIRCLE: ON THE HIP

Continue to work on your core muscles as you switch the
Circle to one arm. Maintain your box and work your upper
arm muscles – your arm works like a hinge as the elbow
pulls the Circle in towards the body, compressing it smaller
and tighter with each repetition.

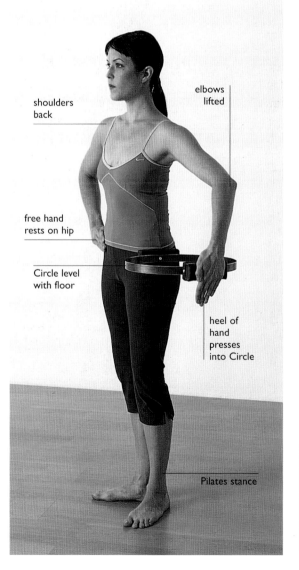

shoulders
back

elbows
lifted

free hand
rests on hip

Circle level
with floor

heel of
hand
presses
into Circle

Pilates stance

Place the Circle to one side, resting it
squarely on the crest of the hipbone.
Exhale to hug the Circle, pulling the
palm towards the hipbone. Squeeze for
3 counts and smoothly release. Repeat
3–5 times with each arm.

HEAD-TO-TOE CHECKLIST

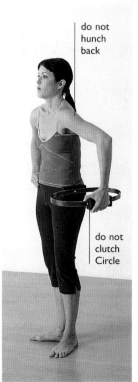

do not
hunch
back

do not
clutch
Circle

• **Place** the Circle on
your hipbone – not on
your waist.
• **Relax** the neck and
shoulders to avoid
contracting the chest.
• **Do not** clutch the pad
of the Circle – the thumb
should remain with the
rest of the fingers.
• **Tighten** the buttocks
but do not tuck your
hips under or push the
pelvis forwards.

MAGIC CIRCLE: AT THE BACK

To isolate the muscles in the back of the arms, we hold the Circle behind us. Maintaining good posture is far more challenging in this position. Contract the Circle while keeping the chest open. At first the Circle may barely move but, with regular practice, your strength will improve.

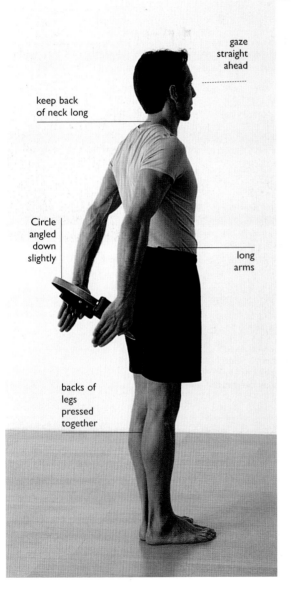

gaze straight ahead

keep back of neck long

Circle angled down slightly

long arms

backs of legs pressed together

Grasp the Circle behind you, tipped slightly downwards. Press the wings down and lengthen the back of the neck. Squeeze the Circle, bringing the entire length of the arms closer together. Hold for 3 counts and release. Repeat 3–5 times.

HEAD-TO-TOE CHECKLIST

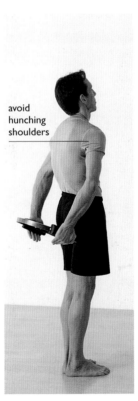

avoid hunching shoulders

- **The Circle** should never touch your body.
- **Keep** the back of the neck long and the gaze straight ahead.
- **Open** the chest. Avoid collapsing the upper body.
- **To avoid** bending the arms or lifting the Circle, think of pressing the upper arms in towards each other as you reach them long.
- **Keep** drawing the navel in and up.

MAGIC CIRCLE: PUMPING

Now we add motion to the previously static exercises. Pump the Circle continuously as you hold the rest of your body solid. Engage your wings, scoop up your navel, and move fluidly.

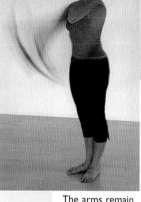

navel scooped up

arms extended

1 Begin with the Circle down low as in Hip Level (*see p166*). Rhythmically pump the Circle for 8 counts, smoothly raising it overhead. Breathe naturally throughout.

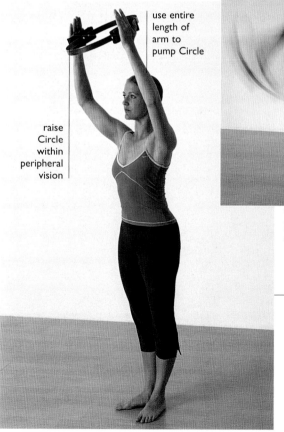

use entire length of arm to pump Circle

raise Circle within peripheral vision

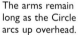

The arms remain long as the Circle arcs up overhead.

2 Reverse the pumping, returning the Circle to your starting position and repeat 3 full sets. This is a moving exercise, so do not pause or stall in any one position. Your posture should remain the same despite the movement of the Circle. Do not allow the upper body to lean back or the hips to press forwards as your arms move up and down.

MAGIC CIRCLE: PLIES

This is the final standing exercise with the Circle. Grow taller as you squeeze the Circle between your legs. This exercise will tone your bottom and inner thighs as well as improve your balance.

1 Stand with your hands on your hips and the Circle between your knees. The feet are in a narrow triangle and the knees are open over the toes. Begin with the knees bent and your spine in one long line from head to tail.

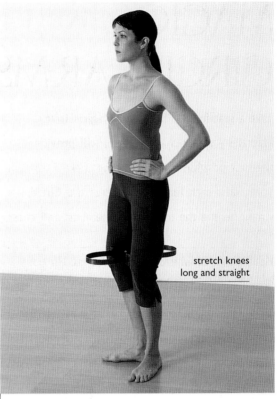

stretch knees long and straight

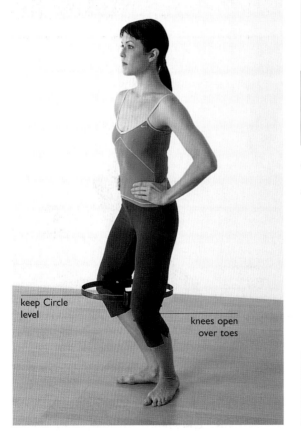

keep Circle level

knees open over toes

2 Straighten your legs, gently squeezing the Circle and rising up taller for 3 counts. Bend your knees to repeat 3–5 times. Tighten the buttocks each time you stretch the knees.

HEAD-TO-TOE CHECKLIST

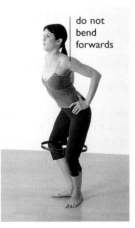

do not bend forwards

• **If you have** weak knees, perform this carefully. You may perform the sitting inner thigh exercise (*right*) as an alternative.

• **Keep** a tall, straight spine. Do not bend forwards or allow your bottom to relax.

• **Bring** the backs of your legs together as you straighten up.

MAGIC CIRCLE: ARMS

Take a seat for the final two Magic Circle exercises – a low chair or stool will provide the best position for performing these. Lengthen your waist each time you squeeze the Circle, strengthening the muscles of the arms and chest.

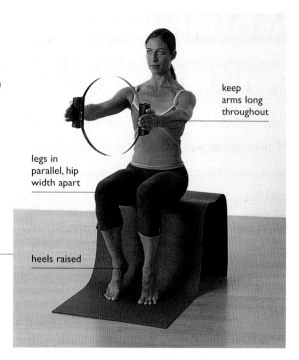

keep arms long throughout

legs in parallel, hip width apart

heels raised

Hold the Circle with outstretched arms. Lift your heels and press the balls of the feet down into the floor. Tighten your bottom, but do not tuck under, as you squeeze the Circle. Hold for 3 counts and slowly release. Repeat 3–5 times.

MAGIC CIRCLE: INNER THIGHS

We conclude the Magic Circle work with a seated inner thigh exercise. Once again, we focus on narrowing the waistline as well as on posture and alignment. With the feet flat on the floor, position the heels as close together as possible.

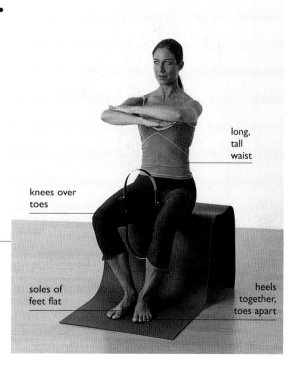

long, tall waist

knees over toes

soles of feet flat

heels together, toes apart

Place the Circle – facing straight out – at the fleshy part of your thighs, just above your knees. Cross your arms over one another from fingertips to elbows. Exhale as you squeeze the Circle and hold for 3 counts. Slowly relax. Repeat 3–5 times.

USEFUL RESOURCES

There are numerous resources for Pilates and Pilates training. If you would like to get started, find a teacher that you feel comfortable with, teaching a style that you feel is appropriate for your level. Always ask how much experience a teacher has had and where they trained. This book describes the authentic Pilates technique, but many different styles exist. Explore the options available to you locally.

GENERAL RESOURCES

For studio listings, teacher training organizations, and Pilates education materials worldwide. Also websites with Pilates-related articles.

Presentation Dynamics Inc.
774 Mays Blvd, Suite 10–143
Incline Village
NV 89451
Tel: (775) 832–8210
Fax: (435) 808–0919
Email: info@bodymind.net
www.bodymind.net
Specializing in Joseph Pilates: matwork, equipment, and exercises.

www.pilates.co.uk
A comprehensive website dedicated to the Pilates method of exercise and providing links to the global Pilates network.

www.pilatesbodyworksintl.com
Information about Pilates studios, other websites, employment opportunities, certification programmes, seminars, educational events, and equipment.

www.classicalpilates.net
Offers Pilates videos demonstrating classical Pilates, including the complete Pilates mat series.

STUDIO REFERRALS AND PROFESSIONAL RESOURCES

Referral source for Pilates teachers and industry professionals.

The PILATESfoundation® UK Limited
80 Camden Road
London E17 7NF
Tel: +44 (0)70–7178–1859
Fax: +44 (0)20–8281–5087
Email: admin@pilatesfoundation.com
www.pilatesfoundation.com

The Pilates Method Alliance
PO Box 370906
Miami
FL 33137–0906
Tel Toll Free: 1–866–573–4945
Email: info@pilatesmethodalliance.org
www.pilatesmethodalliance.org

The New York Pilates Studio ® of Australia
Cynthia Lochard, Director
Suite 12, Level 4
46–58 Holt Street
Surry Hills
NSW 2010
Australia
Phone: (02) 9698–4689, Fax: (02) 9698–4689
Email: contact@pilatesm.com.au
www.pilatesm.com.au

The Pilates Institute of Australasia Pty Ltd
PO Box 1046
North Sydney, NSW 2059
Australia
Tel: (02) 8920–2622, Fax: (02) 8920–2633
Email: info@pilates.net
www.pilates.net

EQUIPMENT
Sources for retail and wholesale equipment.
(Note: Hugger Mugger supplied the mats used
throughout the book, sweatyBetty supplied the
clothing, and Peak Body Systems supplied the
Magic Circle.)

Gratz Industries Inc.
13–06 Queens Plaza South
Long Island City
NY 11101
Tel: (718) 361–7774
www.pilates-gratz.com

Hugger Mugger Yoga Products
3937 So 500 W
Salt Lake City
Utah 84123
Tel: (800) 473–4888
Fax: (801) 268–2629
www.huggermugger.com

also available at:
Hugger Mugger Ltd
12 Roseneath Place
Edinburgh EH9 1JB
Tel: 0131–221–9977
Email: yme@ednet.co.uk,
www.yoga.co.uk

Peak Body Systems
5425 Airport Blvd, Suite 103
Boulder, CO 80301
Tel: (303) 998–1531, Toll Free: (800) 925–3674
www.peakbodysystems.com

sweatyBetty
Tel: 0800–169–3889
Email: info@sweatybetty.com
www.sweatybetty.com
Women's sportswear retailer with shops located at:

833 Fulham Road, London SW6 5HQ
Tel: 020–7751–0228, Fax: 020–7751–0229

5 Kensington Church Street, London W8 4LD
Tel: 020–7937–5523, Fax: 020–7937–5490

110 Westbourne Grove, London W2 5RU
Tel: 020–7751–0228, Fax: 020–7751–0229

TO CONTACT ALYCEA UNGARO
Tribeca Bodyworks
Pilates Center of New York
177 Duane Street
New York, NY 10013
Tel: (212) 625–0777
Fax: (212) 625–0030
Email: PilatesNYC@aol.com
www.tribecabodyworks.com

TO CONTACT ROMANA KRYZANOWSKA
Drago's Gym
Romana Kryzanowska – Master Teacher
50 West 57th Street, 6th Floor
New York, NY 10019
Tel: (212) 757–0724

INDEX

ACKNOWLEDGMENTS

AUTHOR'S ACKNOWLEDGMENTS

As with all artistic endeavours, special thanks must be expressed to the people who come together and create something from nothing. I am extremely grateful to the team at Dorling Kindersley, who toiled day and night to make this project materialize in spite of the ocean separating us. Thanks in particular to Tracy Killick for her vision, Irene Lyford for her ability to string words together seamlessly, and to Russell Sadur for his unique ability to capture movement through the lens of a camera. I would also like to thank Mary-Clare Jerram, Gillian Roberts, Jenny Jones, Sara Robin, Kenny Grant, and Nina Duncan.

My personal support system was unfaltering and extraordinarily tolerant during the months of writing. Thanks to my husband Robert, my dear mother, my wonderful friends, and the entire crew at Tribeca Bodyworks. Special recognition must be given to the models who survived hours of torturous posing, as well as to Bob Liekens for his expert technical input.

Finally, a warm thank you to Katie Allen for suggesting this project in the first place, and to Romana Kryzanowska for a decade of training.

PUBLISHER'S ACKNOWLEDGMENTS

Dorling Kindersley would like to thank photographer Russell Sadur and his assistant, Nina Duncan; models Kathy Buccellato, Jeff Elsass, Elizabeth Jay, and Collette Stewart; Grant le Duc at Eagles Nest Daylight Studio, New York; Bruce James Group, New York, for set building; Tamami Mihara and Kaori Yanagida for models' hair and makeup.

Special thanks to the staff at sweatyBetty, 883 Fulham Road, London SW6 5HQ for the loan of Nike clothing (see p173 for further contact details); to Hugger Mugger Yoga Products for supplying the mats used in the photography throughout this book (see p173 for contact details); and to Peak Body Systems for supplying the Magic Circle (see p173 for contact details).

Finally, Dorling Kindersley would also like to thank Lynn Bresler for compiling the Index and Cheryl Dubyk-Yates for picture research.

PHOTOGRAPHIC ACKNOWLEDGMENTS

The publisher would like to thank the following for their kind permission to reproduce their photographs:
I.C. Rapoport, 1961: pp9, 10
All other images © Dorling Kindersley.
For further information see: www.dkimages.com

All the quotations used in the Introduction to this book are by Joseph Pilates

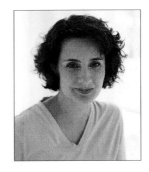

ABOUT THE AUTHOR

Alycea Ungaro, a licensed physical therapist, is the founder and director of the Pilates Center of New York – Tribeca Bodyworks, New York's largest Pilates centre. Alycea began studying Pilates at the age of 14 while attending New York City Ballet's prestigious School of American Ballet. After a decade of increasing proficiency as a student of the Pilates method, Alycea became a certified Pilates instructor under the tutelage of Master instructor Romana Kryzanowska, Joseph Pilates' chosen successor. In 1995 she established Tribeca Bodyworks, a studio dedicated to teaching the classic techniques developed by Joseph Pilates. Here she has personally trained Madonna, Uma Thurman, Matthew Modine, and many others. Alycea authored her first book, *Portable Pilates,* in 2000. She currently lives in New York City with her husband and two daughters.